Intra-articular and Allied Injections

Intra-articular and Allied Injections

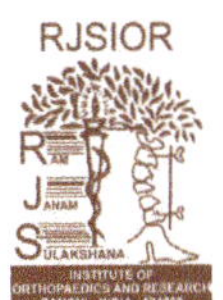

Fourth Edition

Sureshwar Pandey
MBBS(Hons) MS(Gen) FICS FIAMS MS(Ortho) FACFAS FACS FNAMS
Professor Emeritus, University of Ranchi
Founder and Founder Director, Charitable GNH Handicapped Children Hospital and
RJS Artificial Limb Centre, Ranchi
Founder and Consultant, Ram Janam Sulakshana
Institute of Orthopaedics and Research, Ranchi, Jharkhand, India
Founder and Emeritus President and Ex-Secretary General, Indian Foot and Ankle Society
[Affiliated to International Federation of Foot and Ankle Societies (IFFAS)]
Founder and Emeritus Editor, The Journal of Foot and Ankle Surgery
Visiting Professor, Universities of Tokyo, Osaka, Teikyo, Adelaide, Flinders,
Ujung Pandang, Singapore
Ex-Chairman, ASIA-CIP (IFFAS)
Founder and Chairman, Ram Janam Sulakshana Pandey Charitable
Cancer Hospital & Research and Rehabilitation Centre, Ranchi
Hon President, Asia-Pacific Society for Foot and Ankle Surgery

- Best Book Award of BOS (2000–2001) for his Book Clinical Orthopaedic Diagnosis, 2nd Edition
- Best Book Award of BOA 2002 for his Unique Books
- Best Book Award (2009–2010) for his Book—The Clubfoot Revisited
- Humanitarian Award of India of IOA – 2019

Anil Kumar Pandey
MBBS CORM PhD(Ortho) MAMS
Director and Consultant
Ram Janam Sulakshana Institute of Orthopaedics and Research (RJSIOR)
Associate Director and Consultant
GNH Handicapped Children Hospital and RJS Artificial Limb Centre
Executive Director and Consultant
Ram Janam Sulakshana Pandey Charitable Cancer Hospital and
Research and Rehabilitation Centre
Ranchi, Jharkhand, India
Consultant—Kiran Centre for Education and Rehabilitation
Varanasi, Uttar Pradesh, India
Consultant—RAHA, Chhattisgarh, India
Reconstructive Surgeon, Rotary International Project, Government of Nigeria
Fifth Edition

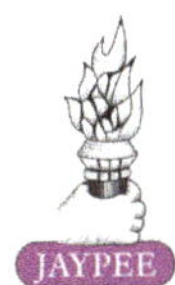

JAYPEE BROTHERS MEDICAL PUBLISHERS
The Health Sciences Publisher
New Delhi | London

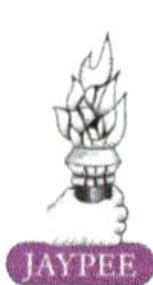

Jaypee Brothers Medical Publishers (P) Ltd

Headquarters
EMCA House
23/23-B, Ansari Road, Daryaganj
New Delhi 110 002, India
Landline: +91-11-23272143
+91-11-23272703, +91-11-23282021
+91-11-23245672
E-mail: jaypee@jaypeebrothers.com

Corporate Office
Jaypee Brothers Medical Publishers (P) Ltd.
4838/24, Ansari Road, Daryaganj
New Delhi 110 002, India
Phone: +91-11-43574357
Fax: +91-11-43574314
E-mail: jaypee@jaypeebrothers.com

Overseas Office
JP Medical Ltd.
83, Victoria Street, London
SW1H 0HW (UK)
Phone: +44-20 3170 8910
E-mail: info@jpmedpub.com

EU GPSR Authorised Representative
Logos Europe, 9 rue Nicolas Poussin
17000, La Rochelle, France
Phone: +33 (0) 6 67 93 73 78
E-mail: Contact@logoseurope.eu

Website: www.jaypeebrothers.com
Website: www.jaypeedigital.com

Inquiries for bulk sales may be solicited at: jaypee@jaypeebrothers.com

Intra-articular and Allied Injections / ***Sureshwar Pandey, Anil Kumar Pandey***
First Edition: 1982
First Japanese Edition: 1987
Second Edition: 2005
American Edition: 2007
Third Edition: 2017
Third Edition: Digital Version 2018
Fourth Edition: **2025**

ISBN: 978-93-5696-636-9

Dedicated to

The sacred memories of my beloved Godly parents

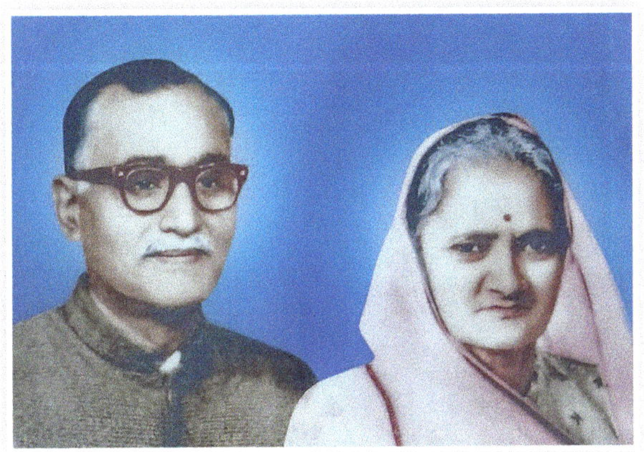

Smt Sulakshana Pandey
and
Pandit Ramjanam Pandey

- *Who were, are, and will always be with me to love, teach, and guide.*
- *Who taught me to persuade my dreams, since nothing is impossible with sincere and devoted efforts.*
- *Who gave me everything, but never even desired to have anything from me.*

Preface

This book appeared as a small booklet in the early 1980s; however, since then itself, it started gaining popularity not only in India but also abroad. The first Japanese edition of this book appeared in 1987. Thence, its American edition was published by McGraw Hill. The American edition was represented in the International Book Fair at Frankfurt, Germany. In this 4th edition, some additions have been made as allied subjects such as "Acupuncture", "Reiki", and "Yoga", since they also impart more or less comparable benefits. In preparing this edition, besides the efforts of my coauthor Dr Anil Kumar Pandey, the fleet of doctors of my family—Dr Pushpa Pandey, Dr Shivam, Dr Pallavi, Dr Sangam, Dr Vaishnavi, Dr Gaurav, Dr Somyanil, Dr Mohan, Adv Shruti and Hitesh Vashistsh, and Dr Satyam—helped us at every step. Dr Madhukar Anand, my co-worker, has exerted a lot in preparing the manuscript and liaisoning with the publisher. He deserves special mention of thanks. Dr Shabana, Ms Mileta Xalxo, Ms Sarita Thapa, and Ms Laxmi Kumari have always been at our help in preparing this book. I frankly admit that my driving forces are the little angels Atharva Pranjal, Adhrit Pranjal, and Yuvraj Harish.

Sureshwar Pandey

Contents

CHAPTER 1

Principles of Intra-articular and Allied Injections

"Change is inevitable, progress is a choice."

—**Dean Lindsay**

CHAPTER OUTLINE

- Mode of action of glucocorticoids
- Immune responses
- Anti-inflammatory properties
- Potency

INTRODUCTION

It is more than five decades from now that Philip Hench and his colleagues introduced the corticosteroids with a lot of fan and fair (triumphal and trumpeted introduction indeed) for managing rheumatoid arthritis at the Mayo clinic in 1949.

In fact, Kendall and Hench in America and Reichstein in Switzerland jointly won the Nobel Prize for the introduction of cortisone, which was used for the first time in 1948 for treating rheumatoid arthritis. Soon after it was observed by Philip Hench and his colleagues at Mayo clinic (1949) that hydrocortisone was active at tissue level in reducing the inflammatory changes. However, now responsible physicians always want to ward off the steroids or wean them off (if it has already being used) as far as possible. Of course, its one use still remains and perhaps will remain (till some harmless substitute comes in the medical arena) universally employed and that is its intra-articular, periarticular and intralesional injections/infiltrations.

The joint aspiration was practiced as early as in 1930s. Perhaps the first intra-articular injections were of formalin and glycerin, lipidol, lactic acid and petroleum jelly which yielded some benefit (Pemberton R 1935; Ropes MW and Bauer W 1953).

Joe Hollander (1951) was the first to introduce the local infiltrative use and intra-articular injection of hydrocortisone acetate to control pain and limit the inflammatory process, whether induced by trauma, collagen arthropathy or crystallopathy or similar conditions. He observed much better clinical response in a series of more than 100,000 hydrocortisone acetate injection in 4,000 patients. Oral use of corticosteroids is very popular with the physicians even general practitioners, but its local use demands a skilled approach, a knowledge placement and careful precautions to avoid infections. The surgeons or rheumatologists or gynecologists or dermatologists or ophthalmologists need to know absolutely where, when, how, why and why not to use it.

Hollander was perhaps one of the first to use compound F (hydrocortisone acetate) into an inflamed joint due to rheumatoid arthritis and had also used prednisolone tertiary butyl acetate to prolong the benefit. Hydrocortisone acetate (an acetate ester of hydrocortisone) is a very fine white odorless crystalline powder and is practically insoluble in water (considerably less soluble than the hydrocortisone in aqueous media). It melts at a temperature of 216–220°C. One gram dissolves in 230 mL of alcohol and 150 mL of chloroform.

The preparation most commonly, effectively and widely used till recently is hydrocortisone tertiary acetate ester of triamcinolone acetinide (TATBA). The chemical formula of hydrocortisone acetate is $C_{23}H_{32}O_6$. The injection available is a sterile suspension of hydrocortisone acetate in sodium chloride solution, containing a dispersing agent.

The usual dose of hydrocortisone acetate for intra-articular injection is 25 mg for an average joint with a variation from 0.5 to 50 mg. Several joints can be injected simultaneously.

MODE OF ACTION OF GLUCOCORTICOIDS

Glucocorticoids diffuse across the cell membrane and form a complex with specific cytoplasmic receptors. These complexes enter the nucleus of the cell, bind to the DNA and stimulate transcription of mRNA and later protein synthesis of various enzymes. On the whole, this is the basic biochemical action of the steroid which accounts for the various and numerous effects after the systemic use.

As such the mode of action of adrenocortical steroids has been mainly discussed around:

1. Immune responses.
2. Anti-inflammatory properties.

However, they also influence the carbohydrate, protein and fat metabolism. They also affect the working of cardiovascular system, skeletal system, skeletal muscles and the central nervous system.

IMMUNE RESPONSES

The mode of immune responses, as yet, has not been clearly defined. They are believed to modify the clinical course of different diseases in which hypersensitivity is believed to play an important role. They do not interfere with the normal mechanism of development of cell-mediated immunity. Probably, they prevent or suppress the inflammatory responses that take place as a consequence of hypersensitivity reactions.

ANTI-INFLAMMATORY PROPERTIES

Researches are still on to understand clearly the anti-inflammatory properties of corticosteroids. However, for the clinicians it is perhaps enough to understand that corticosteroids inhibit the inflammatory responses, whether the inciting agent is radiant, mechanical, chemical, infectious or immunological. It must be borne in mind that there is only suppression of the inflammatory effect, while the underlying causes of the diseases remain unaffected. It is this property of corticosteroids that provides them almost unique potential for therapeutic disaster. Hence, the epitomized remark, at times, stands true that corticosteroids, if misused, permit a patient to walk slowly all the way to the autopsy room. However, the recent works in more detail have projected variable positive thinking about the role of intra-articular corticosteroids.

Corticosteroids exert their anti-inflammatory action by interrupting the inflammatory and immune cascade at several levels including: impairment of antigen opsonization, interference with inflammatory cell adhesion and migration through vascular endothelium, interruption of cell-cell communication by alteration of release or antagonism of cytokines (interleukin-1), impairment of leukotriene and prostaglandin synthesis, inhibition of production of neutrophil superoxide, metalloprotease and metalloprotease activator (plasminogen activator) and decreased immunoglobulin synthesis (Gaffney et al. 1995).

Intra-articular steroids, probably, reduce the number of lymphocytes, macrophages and mast cells, which in turn reduces phagocytosis, lysosomal enzyme release and the release of inflammatory mediators (Snibbe and Gambardella 2005). Thus inflammation is reduced, especially due to reductions in the release of interleukin-1, leukotrienes and prostaglandins (Uthman et al. 2003) and the pain is relieved.

Against earlier reported that corticosteroids injections may suppress cartilage proteoglycan synthesis, worsen cartilage lesion or even cause degenerative lesion in normal cartilage (Raynauld 1999), recent reports have shown that low dose intra-articular corticosteroids (sufficient to suppress catabolism) normalized proteoglycan synthesis and significantly reduced the incidence and severity of cartilage erosions and osteophyte formation (Raynauld JP et al. 2003). In humans, repeated corticosteroid injection in knees of patients with chronic arthritis presented no evidence of destruction or accelerated deterioration (Friedman and Moore, 1980).

The local or intra-articular injection of the corticosteroids does not appear to have significant systemic effects. However, it does not mean that it is all full proof. Slowly there may be a gross damage of the articular cartilage following injudicious repeated use of intra-articular corticosteroids.

The local mode of action is again not clearly defined. Though pioneers have devoted their time and mind to illustrate the exact mode of action of intra-articular hydrocortisone acetate and allied substance (in appendix before bibliography) the controversy still exists. Kantrowitz et al. (1975) suggested that the anti-inflammatory property of corticosteroid emanate from their capacity to inhibit production of prostaglandin (a potent mediator of inflammatory response) in the synovium.

Clinical effects of suppression of nonspecific inflammation and reduction of swelling and pain to varying extent have been noticed in most of the cases with intra-articular injection of the corticosteroids. However, in certain cases it appears as only a palliative therapy and at another few occasions it proves to be ineffective.

It has been noticed that at times even a placebo injection into the joint or even just pricking into the joint helps in relieving the chronic pain to varying extent. This may be explained, more or less on the comparable lines of using electrical stimulation and acupuncture to relieve the chronic pain. Probably, they act by closing a hypothetical GATE in the spinal cord, thereby blocking pain stimuli from reaching the brain. Puncturing stimulates small nerve fibers sending impulses through the OPEN GATE that registers in brain as acute pain. When the signals reach the central biasing mechanism of the brainstem, they trigger counter impulses, which travel down the spinal cord and close the GATE against the chronic pain. However, this is just a hypothesis. Various research works, being done to find the effective ways and means of tackling the problem of pain, point to a new attractive approach basing upon the opposite principles of stimulating the inhibitory systems. Of course, it is too early to provide an objective evaluation of such possibilities. Low doses of intra-articular steroids have been noticed to reduce the size, severity and progression of both, lesions of the cartilage and osteophyte formation (William 1985, Pelletier et al. 1994).

Though Moskowitz et al. (1985) and Behrens (1975) have raised the possibilities of adverse effects of intra-articular corticosteroids on the articular cartilage, varying benefits from such injections cannot be denied (Freidman 1980, Dieppe et al. 1980, Pandey 1982), rather its judicious use can always be beneficial (Pandey 1982).

It has been a general tendency to use intra-articular steroids in late stage of osteoarthritis or other similar arthritic conditions, but this strategy needs to be changed in light of the experimental evidences, which indicate that intra-articular steroids exert a chondroprotective effect—it is probably by the suppression of stromelysin synthesis, a metalloprotease implicated in osteoarthritic cartilage degradation. However, though pain relief by intra-articular corticosteroids can be dramatic, its long-term chondroprotective effects need further authentication.

Hydrocortisone the natural hormone, being too much soluble was found to disperse too quickly, and thus, could not leave its prolonged effects locally. Hence, its chemically improved ester form hydrocortisone acetate

($C_{23}H_{32}O_6$), the primary alcohol group of C_{23} being the one esterified, was developed and found to be suitable.

It is considerably less soluble than hydrocortisone in aqueous media, rather for all practical purposes hydrocortisone acetate may be taken as insoluble in water. It melts at a temperature of 216–220°C. One gram dissolves in 230 mL of alcohol and 150 mL of chloroform. When prepared in microcrystalline form and mixed with other agents it forms a stable suspension, which can be injected locally where it remains deposited for several weeks, gradually releasing the hydrocortisone to produce its anti-inflammatory effects for longer period. The successful attempt to restore the comfort and mobility of rheumatoid affected joints by local injection of hydrocortisone acetate (compound F) into the inflamed joint was by Hollander, the Philadelphia rheumatologist in 1951. He used prednisolone tertiary butyl acetate to prolong the benefit. McCarty, the Hollander's colleague rheumatologist in Philadelphia, showed that the very long-lasting synthetic corticosteroid derivatives, especially triamcinolone hexacetonide (TATBA or THA), could produce remarkable and lasting remissions of the rheumatoid arthritis effects when given as multiple injections at certain intervals, especially in smaller joints (e.g., in hands). He equated the result to the 'medical synovectomy'. With the pioneering work of these two rheumatologists ushered the art and science of local injection therapy for the rheumatic disorders. Of course, the experiences of ameliorating pain by injecting local anesthetic agents into and around the painful spots in the muscles and painful ligaments in the sprains have definite role in establishing the local injection therapy for rheumatoid disorders and allied conditions.

Gradually, there has been great swing in favor of injecting methyl-prednisolone acetate (chemical name being 6-methyl-delta-1-hydro-cortisone) in place of hydrocortisone acetate, wherever it is indicated. It is 6-methyl derivative of prednisolone. Methylprednisolone acetate possess the general properties of the glucocorticoid methylprednisolone, but is less soluble, and therefore, less readily metabolized. Thus, after injection into various sites its action is prolonged. It is more or less white odorless crystalline powder which melts at about 215°C with slight decomposition and is practically insoluble in water. Its molecular formula is "$C_{22}H_{30}O_5$" and has the molecular weight of 374.46.

Like other glucocorticoids, methylprednisolone causes profound and varied metabolic effects. These compounds have also been seen to modify the body's immune response to diverse stimuli.

The rate of systemic absorption of an intra-articular corticosteroid is proportionate to the solubility of the compound. More insoluble compounds are better suited for intra-articular use, since the local duration of action is prolonged and the chances of systemic absorption remain minimum. Methyl-prednisolone acetate and the triamcinolone hexacetonide are widely used for intra-articular injection, followed by the use of triamcinolone acetonide.

POTENCY

The potency of 4 mg of methylprednisolone can be obtained from 4.4 mg of methylprednisolone acetate. The anti-inflammatory effect of 20 mg of hydrocortisone is available from the 4.4 mg of methylprednisolone acetate. Mineralocorticoid activity of methylprednisolone is minimal. 200 mg of methylprednisolone is equivalent to 1 mg of desoxycorticosterone. Intra-articular injection of Dysprosium-165-ferric hydroxide macroaggregates has been used for medical synovectomy and has been proved to be an effective treatment for chronic rheumatoid synovitis of the knee with minimum radiographic evidence of lesion of bone and cartilage (stage I or stage II radiographic changes).

The low rates of systemic spread of the isotope offer a definite advantage over previously used agents for radiation synovectomy, e.g., chemical such as osmic acid and alkylating agents, e.g., (thiotepa and nitrogen mustard); several radionuclides in colloidal or particulate form, e.g., yttrium-90, gold-198, ebrium-169, rhenium-186 and phosphorus-32 (Sledge et al. 1987). Dysphrosium-165 is a rare earth element with a half-life of 2.3 hours. It decays mainly by beta emissions. The maximum extent of penetration of the beta emission into the soft tissue is 5.7 mm, which probably approximates the entire synovial lining of the joint.

CHAPTER 2

How Frequently to Inject Corticosteroid?

"Take time to deliberate, but when the time for action has arrived, stop thinking and go in."

—Napoleon Bonaparte

CHAPTER OUTLINE

- Reasons for injecting between 2 and 4 weeks, and utmost 6 weeks
- Why should intra-articular corticosteroid not be given more frequently?
- Whether intra-articular corticosteroid should be given as cocktail or alone?
- Role of hyaluronidase

In case of hydrocortisone acetate, since the preparation used is in acetate form of suspension, there has to be slow dispersal of the drug. It is rather difficult to pinpoint the number of injections required for a particular case, but a working line can be projected on the basis of experiences.

Probably, the most suitable schedule will be at 3 weeks interval and never to be repeated in <2 weeks. Even the intervals of 4–6 weeks has been found to be equally suitable and effective in several instances. Hence, the working rule should be to keep an interval of not <2 weeks and not >6 weeks. It has been observed that if three consecutive injections are not effective in ameliorating the patients condition to appreciable extent, it will be probably not effective even with more injections. In such conditions, considering the possible hazards of intra-articular hydrocortisone acetate injections it should be abandoned henceforth. In giving bi-weekly injections, the moment symptoms are completely relieved, no further injection should be given. Even if the symptoms are not completely relieved by up to five, weekly or fortnightly, injections, further injection should not be given. It has been observed that the cases which are going to respond, usually show adequate response at the very first properly given injection. If there is no appreciable response when injection into the synovial space is given as determined by the aspiration of synovial fluid, repeated injections may be futile, rather may be even harmful. The interval between two pricks may be placed between 2 and 4 weeks. Perhaps, beyond 4 weeks, relief obtained after the first injection may not be adequately carried over. Of course, in certain circumstances where, per chance, arthrotomy happened to be performed even after several months of intra-articular injections, the chalky deposits of hydrocortisone acetate could be demonstrated at different places in the joint, especially near the attachments of intra-articular ligaments (e.g., cruciate ligament in knee, ligamentum teres in head of femur) or at the margins of capsular attachment.

James et al. (1996) observed that in most patients of osteoarthritis, corticosteroid injections provide pain relief but it may not last for more than a few weeks. However, this observation is true in very less number of cases, rather many remain pain-free for more longer period (several months to year or even more sometimes).

WHY SHOULD INTRA-ARTICULAR CORTICOSTEROID NOT BE GIVEN MORE FREQUENTLY?

Perhaps there is hardly any general toxicity of local corticosteroid injections, but the local damaging effects over the structures of the joints have been noticed. **Neuropathic-like changes** on the structures of the joints, especially in the knee (most frequent site of intra-articular injection of corticosteroids) have been reported. Whether the changes are subsequent to prolonged repeated injections of local anesthetics or local injection of corticosteroid or both, is matter of controversy. However, adequate experimental evidences have been gathered to blame corticosteroid injections to be responsible for neuropathic like changes in the joints.

The overall economic factor should also not be ignored as patients have to come from varying distance to proper place for intra-articular injections. In such circumstances, there does not appear any logic in asking the patient to come repeatedly if the initial response is not adequate. In the absence of early adequate response, the patient should not be kept hanging on wishful thinkings. Rather than repeating intra-articular corticosteroid injection the surgeon should resort to appropriate surgical intervention, if needed.

WHETHER INTRA-ARTICULAR CORTICOSTEROID SHOULD BE GIVEN AS COCKTAIL OR ALONE?

In joints having easily definable space, corticosteroid may be injected alone. However, a cocktail of corticosteroid, lidocaine hydrochloride and hyaluronidase have been advocated to be more effective, when it is to be given in the soft tissues rather than into the synovial spaces. The hyaluronidase undoubtedly helps in easily spreading the corticosteroid. It seems to have no other advantage. However, it is a foreign protein and allergy may develop if the injections are repeated and it should be omitted in repeated use.

Hyaluronidase is a naturally occurring enzyme. It is found in the human (and mammals) semen, snake venom and certain bacteria. For clinical use it is purified so as to remove most of the inert material. The resultant solution is sterilized and freeze-dried into a white or yellowish white powder.

It has a temporary and reversible depolymerizing action on the hyaluronic acid and chondroitin sulfate polysaccharides, which are normally present in the intercellular matrix of connective tissues. The intercellular cement is, thus, broken down, thereby reducing its viscocity and rendering the tissues more permeable, which facilitates in rapid dispersal of the adjoining solution (e.g., local anesthetic, corticosteroid solution, transfusion fluid, etc.). It also promotes the reabsorption of excess fluid and blood from the tissues.

Hyaluronidase has been widely used in various fields (especially as an adjuvant to local anesthetic agents) such as obstetric, ophthalmology, dentistry, anorectal and plastic surgery. In orthopedics, its use has been very limited (e.g., for ganglion aspiration).

The standard dose is 1,500 units of hyaluronidase injection.

The lidocaine is for local analgesia. In such circumstances, the volume of injections should also be taken care of and the cocktail must be accordingly adjusted.

In joints like metacarpophalangeal, interphalangeal and temporomandibular ones, only hydrocortisone or other corticosteroids may be injected. But 0.5–1 mL of local anesthetic may be added to act as a vehicle for smaller amount of drug. This also acts as local anesthetic to some extent.

In joints, where surface area is more tortuous or intervened with more watershades, e.g., shoulder, hip and spinal joints, the cocktail of local anesthetic and corticosteroid is suitable. It has been the practice in a few hands to infiltrate a local anesthetic first, and to leave the needle there in the space. Subsequently, the cocktail or corticosteroid alone is pushed into. This procedure is not always needed except for the beginners where the joint space may not be reached in a single direct prick. It carries a potential drawback that the joint space is communicating to the exterior threatening to carry the airborne infecting agents into the joints. Further, manipulating the top of the open needle-end with bare fingers also carries the potential risk of contamination. Hence, wherever desired, it is better to prepare a cocktail earlier, load into the syringe and push directly into the desired space. The pain of prick will be always there, even for infiltrating the local anesthetic prior to injecting the corticosteroid.

Many other preparations have been injected into the joints (in appendix before bibliography). Others, which are essentially radioactive or chemical cauterizing agents, are of limited specialized value and require special facilities and expertise.

Substances such as orgotein (pharmaceutical form of the bovine enzyme Cu-Zn superoxide dismutase), radiation synovectomy (dysprosium-165 hydroxide macroaggregate, yttrium-90 silicate), dextrose prolotherapy, silicone, saline lavage, saline injection without lavage, analgesic agents (bupivicaine, morphine), nonsteroidal anti-inflammatory drug (NSAIDs) [tenoxicam, indoprofen, phenylbutazone, glucosamine, somatostatin, sodium pentosan polysulfate (NAPP)], chloroquine, mucopolysaccharide polysulfuric acid ester, lactic acid solution, 10% dextrose, cytostatica (thiotepa, azetepa, osmium acid) have been investigated as potentially therapeutic in the treatment of arthritic joints.

CHAPTER 3

How to Inject?

"Plans are nothing, planning is everything."

—Dwight D Eisenhower

CHAPTER OUTLINE

- Word of caution
- Localization of the site of the injection

Perhaps no one can predict in which particular case corticosteroid (or substitute) is going to provide relief, but everyone must take it for granted that even a slight negligence on the part of the injecting hand can spoil the joint for years or even forever.

Before injecting ask yourself a few questions:

- Does this joint require any injection into it?
- Is the surface over and around the joints free from infective focus?
- Are you competent enough to invade into the virginity of the joint?
- Is your patient free from diabetes?
- Are the syringe, needle and other equipments/instruments thoroughly sterilized?

WORD OF CAUTION

Let us be very honest, it is not certain in most of the cases where we are injecting hydrocortisone acetate or other steroids that we are definitely going to give relief to the patient but it is almost certain that we can always be culprit of introducing infective organism with devastating effects, perhaps irreversible in most of the cases, unless we are truly aseptic in our procedure. Let us not rob the patient of the residual utility of his joints, only with an uncertain attempt to suppress his painful stimuli. This does not mean that one should stop the corticosteroid injection, rather one must use it but with a flash of caution before every prick.

LOCALIZATION OF THE SITE OF THE INJECTION

Since the point of injection must not be touched after cleaning, it is always essential to mark the injection spot prior to cleaning. Except for the bigger joint (e.g., knee, where joint line can be delineated easily at the either side of the ligamentum patellae) it is better to pinpoint the injection spot by prior marking. It is further important while injecting into soft tissue, e.g., for **lateral epicondylitis, golfer's elbow**.

Two methods can be adopted. Using the skin pencil, the joint line/or the point of maximum tenderness can be marked by cross point or thumbnail can be used to pinpoint the spot, by producing a dent, which remains visible even after washing and cleaning the area for injecting.

A reference point can also be selected which can be palpated by clean index fingertip, and the needle can be pushed at the nearby previously selected spot in relation to the reference point which is NOT touched at all after thorough cleaning—e.g., in knee joint, index finger tip of left hand can be placed in the infrapatellar fossa on lateral side, if injection has to be given through medial infrapatellar fossa or vice-versa. Similarly, by locating the posterior angle of acromion process, the shoulder joint can be injected through a point just inferior to it without touching it.

It has been observed that even in expert hands the proper joint space and targeted point for injections, are likely to be missed or misplaced in notable number of cases. Hence, now it is being advised that as far as possible the injection should be given under fluoroscopic control.

CHAPTER 4

Indications of Corticosteroid Injection

"Whatever is worth doing is not worth overdoing."

—Helen Mc Horstmann and Eugene E Black

CHAPTER OUTLINE

- Definite indications of corticosteroid injection
- Relative indications of corticosteroid injections
- Tendons (mostly around the tendon cautiously, and very rarely into the tendons)
- Ligaments
- Fibrofatty nodules
- Peripheral nerves
- Resistant (nonspecific or at times specific) backache
- Skin conditions
- Ophthalmic condition
- Gynecological conditions
- Reflex sympathetic dystrophy syndrome (RSDS)
- Trial indications

It has become a very common fashion to prescribe intra or periarticular or intra/peritendinous injections of corticosteroids. We may not be blamed for the statement that in conditions where we are not able to assign any specific cause, and especially if we are not able to allay the patient of the pain, corticosteroid becomes an important feature of our prescription. Should we label it as a nonspecific chemotherapeutic agent for such conditions? This version has a base, because in several nonspecific painful conditions, corticosteroid infiltration does work. Patients get relieved of the symptoms, while the proper ailment remains undiagnosed. However, there are definite indications for its infiltrations. At several places, it is used empirically and at frequent occasions it is a 'hit and miss' prescription.

Local corticosteroid therapy is a very precious therapeutic aid in rheumatology. Awareness and respect of its indications, contraindications and risks by the clinicians lead to very successful use of local corticosteroids in optimal conditions with minimal complications. However, in rheumatoid arthritis concurrent medical management accelerates the recovery. When the systemic gold therapy is contemplated even then local/intra-articular corticosteroid therapy should be considered.

Clear indications for intra-articular injection have not been charted out. However, workable indications may be put as follows: Though not beyond controversy, new studies are showing that inta-articular injections may be helpful in the management of postoperative pain, particularly when opiates are used.

DEFINITE INDICATIONS OF CORTICOSTEROID INJECTION

Convenient sites for intra-articular injection are the knee, ankle, wrist, elbow, shoulder, phalangeal, sternoclavicular and acromioclavicular joints. Difficulty is experienced in injecting into the hip joint. Anatomically, inaccessible joints, such as spinal joints and the joints devoid of synovial space, e.g., sacroiliac joints are also difficult to be injected exactly.

Clinical conditions where corticosteroid injections are definitely indicated:

1. Degenerative arthrosis of joint—primary or secondary.
2. Rheumatoid arthritis of joints—usually as an adjuvant to other appropriate medical and physical management.
3. Psoriatic arthropathy.
4. Peripheral synovial swelling of ankylosing spondylitis and of **Reiter's syndrome**.
5. Synovial structures (e.g., in joints, tendon sheath, bursae) are definite target, where local injection therapy prove useful. However, it should be avoided in uric acid gout, for which more effective treatments are available. Of course, in acute gouty arthritis it has been found to be useful.
6. **Post-traumatic stiffness of the joint.**
7. Post-immobilization stiffness of the joint.
8. Periarthritis shoulder. In frozen shoulder corticosteroid injections along with exercises produce significant improvement.
9. **Nonspecific fibrous ankylosis.**
10. Intra-articular fractures—after aspiration of hemarthrosis—injection should be given—cautiously and only once.
11. **Extra-articular tennis-elbow (lateral epicondylitis of humerus).**
12. **Golfer's-elbow (medial epicondylitis of humerus).**
13. **de-Quervain's disease.**
14. Apophysitis, e.g., **Osgood-Schlatter disease, calcaneal apophysitis.**

While targeting to inject certain zone/structure or/joint, there may be flowing of the injected fluid into the communicating pouches or sheaths or elsewhere. Sometimes there are naturally occurring communications such as those often found between the ankle joint and neighbouring tendon sheaths. Sometimes adventitious communications exist such as those developed in the shoulder region, e.g., in rheumatoid arthritis when the glenohumeral joint and subacromial bursae join together. At times synovial cysts develop near joints, where the communication is usually valvular, when the injected material flows into the synovial cyst but the reverse is not true. In these conditions too, other conservative methods of treatment must be exhausted earlier. In degenerative arthritis, especially that of knee, there is definitive role of intra-articular corticosteroid injection. Other intra-articular substances such as orgotein, radiation synovectomy, dextrose prolotherapy, silicone, saline lavage, saline injection without lavage, analgesic agents, nonsteroidal anti-inflammatory drugs, glucosamine, somatostatin, sodium pentosan polysulphate, chloroquine, mucopolysaccharide polysulphuric acid ester, lactic acid solution and thiotepa cytostatica have been tried as potentially therapeutic agent in the treatment of osteoarthritic joints. Recent observations have indicated that in primary osteoarthritis of knee, intra-articular Hylan G-F_{20} treatment is effective for pain, disability and improving functional capacity. Low dose of intra-articular steroids reduce the size, severity and progression of both lesions of the cartilage and osteophyte formation (Williams 1985, Pelletier et al. 1994). Even though there are possibilities of adverse effects on articular cartilage after repeated injections, its judicious use is mostly beneficial.

The strategy to use intra-articular steroids in late stages of osteoarthritis should be changed in the light of recent experimental evidences, which indicates that intra-articular steroids exert a chondroprotective effect probably by suppression of stromelysin synthesis—a metalloprotease implicated in osteoarthritic cartilage degradation (Pelletier 1989). However, though pain relief by intra-articular steroids can be dramatic, its long-term chondroprotective effects need further authentification.

The overall review of the medical literature reflects that in osteoarthritis corticosteroids and hyaluronic acid are widely used in patients who have not responded to other therapeutic modalities. As a practical approach for a joint (like knee) with effusion, steroid injection should be considered after aspiration of effusion, while in symptomatic dry joint hyaluronic acid approach should be useful.

RELATIVE INDICATIONS OF CORTICOSTEROID INJECTIONS

Conditions have to be picked out from the list given below depending upon the earlier response to other available therapeutic and conservative methods.

TENDONS (MOSTLY AROUND THE TENDON CAUTIOUSLY, AND VERY RARELY INTO THE TENDONS)

The objective is to bathe the tendon (not to infiltrate it) in conditions like:

1. Tenosynovitis.
2. Peri-tendinitis.
3. Tendinitis (not more than two injections, since tendons are liable to rupture after repeated injections).
4. Post-traumatic adhesions in and around tendons.
5. Ganglion in relation to tendon.
6. Tendon involvement in collagen disorders.
7. Post-operative after tendon repair to avoid adhesions—one or two injections only.
8. Reconstruction or substitution of tendon.
9. Early xanthomatous affection of tendon
10. To hasten the recovery from pain and other effects on the joint due to immobilization and/or operation (e.g., plaster cast, traction, arthroplasty).

LIGAMENTS

In most of the places where joint is infiltrated, ligaments (coming in the way) are also infiltrated but at places they may require specific infiltrations, e.g.,

1. Partial avulsion of ligaments leading to pain.
2. Pellegrini-Stieda disease.
3. Strained or sprained ligaments of a joint.
4. Post-traumatic adhesions of the ligaments.
5. Fibrotic nodule in relation to a ligament.
6. Collagen disorder affecting the ligaments.
7. Nonspecific inflammation of the ligaments **(e.g., plantar fasciitis)**.

FIBROFATTY NODULES

Fibrofatty nodules in relation to or even quite distant from the joint have been blamed as a triggering point for some painful conditions (sometimes quite unexplainable). In many cases, they do respond to corticosteroid infiltration.

PERIPHERAL NERVES

Empirically along (perineural zone/sheath and intraneural) the main peripheral nerve or its branches in:

1. **Hansen's neuritis.**
2. **Post-traumatic perineural adhesions or adhesive neuritis.**
3. **Painful neuromas.**
4. **Nonspecific peripheral neuritis.**

5. **Meralgia paresthetica.**
6. Radiculitis—mostly following degenerative rupture of disc or altered joint conditions.
7. **Entrapment neuropathy.**

RESISTANT (NONSPECIFIC OR AT TIMES SPECIFIC) BACKACHE

Resistant (specific or at times nonspecific) backache, a truly unsolved problem, does respond to infiltration of corticosteroid (mostly without any true explanation). It may be given as local infiltration at the most tender spot, into the tender and/or triggering nodule, or as epidural injections (also see the chapter on "Spine").

SKIN CONDITIONS

Local corticosteroid infiltration has been reported to have a definite role in certain skin conditions such as:

1. **Disseminated lupus erythematosus.**
2. Eczematous conditions.
3. Keloid.
4. Nonspecific dermatitis.
5. Leucoderma.
6. **Hard and soft corn.**
7. Alopecia.

Wound healing is a complex physiological process which can be considered and grouped into three phases: inflammation fibroblast proliferation and remodeling wherein abundant extracellular matrix is degraded and immature type Hi collagen is modified into type I collagen. Excessive scars forms as a result of aberrations in this physiologic wound healing process and may arise following any insult to the deep dermis. Excessive scarring leads hypertrophic scars and keloids.

Excessive scarring looks unesthetic and disfiguring. If it is around any joint, it may be disabling keloid and hypertrophic scar usually occurs in second and third decade of both sexes. Hypertrophic scar usually occurs in all races and all skin types. However, keloids are found more in dark skinned people of African descents.

Histologically hypertrophic scars and keloids contain mainly fine well-organized wavy type III collagen oriented parallel to the epidermal surface with abundant nodules containing myofibroblasts large extracellular collagen filaments and plentiful acidic mucopolysaccharides.

Keloid tissue, mostly composed of disorganized type I and III collagen patient complain pain, pruritis and contractures.

Management of hypertrophic scars and keloids includes occlusive dressings, compression therapy, intralesional steroids injection, excision,

Radiation therapy, LASER therapy, interferon therapy. Intralesional steroid injections have been used since mid 1960s.

It has been concluded that corticosteroid injections with steroid ointment application following keloid or hypertrophic scar excision help in reducing the recurrence rate.

OPHTHALMIC CONDITION

Corticosteroid infiltration has been used in corneal ulcer to prevent scar. For the same purpose it has also been used in post-operative or post-traumatic ophthalmic conditions.

GYNECOLOGICAL CONDITIONS

A cocktail consisting of hydrocortisone acetate 1 cc and water for injection 9 cc plus crystalline penicillin/streptomycin plus hyaluronidase has been used earlier for hydrotubation in cases of tubal blockage, which has been replaced nowadays by instillation of placentrex. Hydrocortisone acetate, sometimes, is given after tubal microsurgery.

It has been given intrafetally in cases of post-maturity due to anencephaly.

REFLEX SYMPATHETIC DYSTROPHY SYNDROME (RSDS)

In managing early stage of post-traumatic RSDS, regional intravenous blocks of a mixture of corticosteroids and lidocaine have been found to be highly effective. It is recommended as the first choice treatment because it is simple, safe and well-tolerated (Tountas et al. 1993).

TRIAL INDICATIONS

For the conditions where no specific explanation for the pain and/or stiffness around the joint or bursa, tendon or ligaments, muscle, bone or subcutaneous tissue is available, a trial local infiltration of corticosteroid cocktail in and around the affected area is recommended. In such circumstances, usually one to two injections should be tried. Depending upon the response further injections may be given.

In osteochondrosis of scaphoid (Preiser's disease), lunate (Kienbock's disease) and navicular (Kohler's disease), trial injections of corticosteroid must be given before embarking on surgery.

In **ischiogluteal bursitis (weaver's bottom)** and epiphysitis of metatarsal **(Freiberg's infarction)** cocktail infiltration may give relief. Similarly, in painful **hallux valgus, hallux rigidus, tailor's bunion** (in varus angulation of the fifth toe) and interdigital neuroma **(Morton's toe)** there may be trial indications of corticosteroid cocktail injection.

Injections of corticosteroids can also provide relief but has been occasionally objected for its effect in causing atrophy of fat and leaving small depigmented patches in the skin, in various bursitis like olecranon bursitis (student's elbow), prepatellar bursitis (housemaid's knee) and other bursitis around the knee joint, aspiration followed by intrabursal injection of corticosteroid cocktail may be effective.

In spastic flat foot, if the spasm is dominating, infiltration of lignocaine into the sinus tarsi gives immediate relief. In such cases, infiltration of long-acting local anesthetic may provide lasting results.

Kumar and Siwach K (2019) have observed that periarticular local infiltration is significantly effective for pain control, barely mobilization and functional recovery in comparison to buprenorphine transdermal patch as observed in patients undergoing total hip and knee arthroplasty. Periarticular local infiltration also reduces the total consumption of analgesics postoperatively with better patient satisfaction.

Contraindications for Local Corticosteroid Therapy

"When it is obvious that the goals cannot be reached, don't adjust the goal, adjust the action taken."

—Confucius

CHAPTER OUTLINE

- General infections

GENERAL INFECTIONS

It is an absolute contraindication to all corticosteroid therapy.

- Localized infective focus (mainly pyogenic) even at a distance from the joint to be infiltrated (e.g., skin, ENT, urinary, pulmonary).
- *Any hemostatic disorder*: If the patient is under anticoagulants, there is possibility of developing hemarthrosis. Further, since blood is an excellent culture medium, there is risk of quick proliferation of infective organisms, if per chance get infilterated. Hence, it is a relative contraindication to local corticosteroid therapy because of the risk of infection.
- *Diabetes*: One must be cautious in diabetic patients. Even when controlled, it can favor post-infiltrative infections. Repeated infiltrations can cause diabetic disequilibrium.
- *Prosthetic replacements*: All periprosthetic corticosteroid therapy should be abandoned.
- Inflammatory processes associated with metabolic disorders, collagen diseases, osteoarthritis and similar conditions may be an indication in carefully selected cases, otherwise it is contraindication. The depth and extent of inflammation and circulatory changes can be assessed by some non-invasive investigative technique, e.g., thermography.
- Severe joint disruption.
- Uncorrected static deformity.
- Severe osteoporosis of bones adjacent to joints.
- Unstable joints.
- Neuropathic joints.

- Traumatic arthritis due to intra-articular fractures.
- A local fracture of total joint forms a contraindication.

Role of Triamcinolone

The American Academy of Orthopedic Surgeons (AAOS) 2021 guidelines on knee osteoarthritis states that intra-articular corticosteroids could provide short-term relief for patients with symptomatic osteoarthritis of knee. In 2019 American College of Rheumatology (ACR)/Arthritis Foundation Guideline for the Management of Osteoarthritis, of the Hand, Hip, and Knee; strongly recommended Intra-articular glucocorticoid injection for the patients with knee and/or hip osteoarthritis with conditionally recommended for patient with knee and/or hip osteoarthritis conditionally recommended for patient with hand osteoarthritis (Sharon LK et al. 2020).

Corticosteroids produce significant anti-inflammatory effects. The most widely used corticosteroids include **Triamcinolone Hexacetonide** (THA), triamcinolone acetonide and methylprednisolone acetate acetomide, betamethasone sodium phosphate and betamethasone acetate. These compounds were developed to reduce undesirable hormonal side effects with less rapid dissipation from the joint. Triamcinolone Hexacetonide is the least water-soluble preparation and thus provides the longest duration of effectiveness within the peripheral joint space,

Triamcinolone Hexacetonide is the hexacetonide salt form of triamcinolone, a synthetic glucocorticoid with immunosuppressive and anti-inflammatory activity.

Chemical name is: 9-fluoro-11b,16a,17,21-tetrahydroxy-pregna-1, 4-diene-3,20-dione cyclic 16,17-acetal with 21-(3,3-dimethylbutyrate).

Molecular formula: $C_{30}H_{41}FO_7$.

Molecular mass: 532.6 g/mol.

Triamcinolone Hexacetonide injectable suspension is indicated for intra-articular or periarticular use in adults and adolescents for the symptomatic treatment of subacute and chronic inflammatory joint diseases.

Mechanism of Action

Triamcinolone Hexacetonide, like other corticosteroids has both significant glucocorticoids, anti-inflammatory and minimal (practically no) mineralocorticosteroid activity (therefore no sodium retention).

The primary mechanism of action may be their ability to inhibit the release of cytokines by immune cells. In human corticosteroids reduce the accumulation of lymphocytes at inflammatory sites by a migratory effect.

Immunosuppressant effect, are generally via effects on T cells.

The effects in the tissue of injection site lasts for a long time (few weeks to several months). Less peak levels of steroids lead to less systemic exposure and toxicity.

CHAPTER 6

Intra-articular Hyaluronic Acid and Platelet-rich Plasma Injection

"Change is the only aspect that never changes. Innovation should become a habit if one has to be consistently successful."

—**Rekha Shelly**

CHAPTER OUTLINE

- Viscosupplementation
- Role of hyaluronic acid in osteoarthritis
- Corticosteroids versus hyaluronic acid
- Platelet-rich plasma injection

In the last decade the role of hyaluronic acid (HA) in the management of osteoarthritis and rheumatoid arthritis has been much emphasized.

Hylans is the generic name of hyaluronate. Hyaluronate is a glucosaminoglycan with a repeating disaccharide structure that is composed of D-glucuronic acid in linkage to N-acetyl-D-glucosamine. Free HA occurs only in laboratory conditions, hence hyaluronate or hyaluronan are recommended terms. Combining 12,500 disaccharide units produces one molecule of hyaluronan with a molecular weight of about 5 million. Hyaluronate is a hydrophilic polysaccharide belonging to the group of glucosaminoglycans. When hydrated it assumes a larger molecular volume, and thus, occupies a large spheroidial domain. The molecular network of hyaluronate is permeable to the molecules which are smaller than the network elements. This network works as a sieve for larger molecules.

The hyaluronan solution possesses both elastic and viscous properties. This elastoviscosity of hyaluronan varies according to motion and shear forces. In presence of slower motion and lower shear forces, the solution behaves like a viscous fluid (which denotes that the mechanical energy is dissipated as heat through the movement of the network), whereas with more rapid motion and higher shear forces, its behavior resembles the features of an elastic body (which means that the mechanical energy is stored in the molecular network). Thus, diluted solutions of hyaluronan of sufficient molecular weight can function as effective lubricant when movements are slow and as shock absorbers when movements are fast.

Synovial fluid permeates the superficial layer of the articular cartilage as well as the intracellular matrix of the synovial tissue and capsule. This effectively fills the collagen matrix of the intracellular space with viscoelastic hyaluronan. The joint movements generate a flow of synovial fluid maintaining a continuous exchange of hyaluronan between the synovial fluid and the intercellular fluid of the joint tissue.

The molecular mass of hyaluronan in a normal joint is about 4–5 million. The theological properties of arthritic synovial fluid are less than that of normal fluid, hence a substance intended for viscosupplementation must have considerably greater elastoviscosity than the synovial fluid present in an arthritic joint. This was achieved by the development of a highly elastoviscous solution composed of two crosslinked hyaluronans.

The healthy human knee contains about 2 mL of synovial fluid. Hyaluronic acid is present in the synovial fluid at a concentration of 2–3 mg/mL. The molecule gets bond to proteoglycan to form macromolecular aggregates. In an arthritic knee, the amount of synovial fluid increases many times and becomes viscous, the concentration of HA is decreased by 30–50% and the molecular size is reduced. These changes markedly decrease the properties of synovial fluid, mainly its shock absorption, dissipation and storage of energy caused by trauma, and lubrication of the protective layer of articular cartilage.

VISCOSUPPLEMENTATION

The concept of viscosupplementation for the joint was developed by Endre A Balazs and his co-workers in 1960s. Viscosupplementation was introduced to solve the problems associated with osteoarthritis of knee by virtue of restoring the concentration of synovial fluid (Peyron 1993) **(Figure 6.1)**.

Viscosupplementation Treatment for Knee Arthritis

Hyaluronic acid injections are recommended for individuals who do not respond well to other treatments. Hyaluronic acid is a natural component of joint fluid, and injections help lubricate the knee joint, reducing friction and pain. A systematic review published in the Journal of Pain Research concluded that hyaluronic acid injections were effective in relieving knee pain in patients with osteoarthritis and improving joint function. The treatment is well-tolerated with minimal side effects.

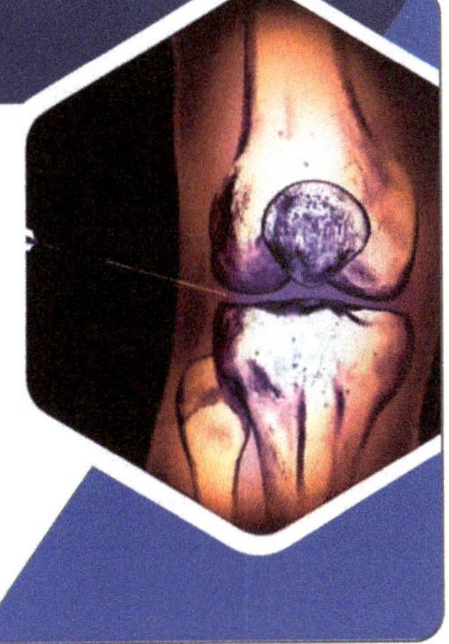

FIG. 6.1: Viscosupplementation—treatment for knee arthritis.

Hylan is an easily deformable gel with fluid-like properties. In 1960s, the development of hyaluronan, derived from human umbilical cord and rooster combs for medical use was begun (Biotrics, Inc., Arlington MA).

Hyaluronate is present in synovial fluid as the major macromolecular component and is responsible for the intrinsic viscoelasticity.

Because of its HA content, joint fluid acts as a viscous lubricant during slow movement of the joint, as in walking and as an elastic shock absorber during rapid movement, as in running. It is considered not only a joint lubricant, but also a physiological factor in the trophic status of cartilage. Hyaluronic acid has a very high water binding capacity. When 1 g of HA is dissolved in physiological saline, it occupies three litres of solution. The estimated total HA in a human knee joint is 4–8 mg (Adams et al. 1995).

Decrease in concentration of hyaluronate is more important factor in the arthropathies than the observed reduction in molecular weight (Balazs EA 1974).

Mechanism of Analgesic Action of Hylan

The exact mechanism of analgesic action of hylan is not known. It is assumed that it acts by virtue of restoring joint homeostasis, which leads to decrease in pain.

The joint motion creates an exertive force, which drives fluid out of joint.

The most significant force, which drives fluid out of a joint is the pressure exerted during joint motion. Lymph channels drain out the fluid in the joint, by which homeostasis is maintained. When the fluid accumulates in joint due to any pathology, the concentration of HA decreases, which leads to a vicious circle. In arthralgia due to pain and increase in fluid volume, the joint movements decrease. In such situation, the injected hylan restores the theological properties of synovial fluid, and thus, may improve the fluid mechanics in the joint, which in turn may improve the joint movements and reduce the pain.

Probably, the ability of hylan to restore joint homeostasis is responsible for its analgesic effects, however, as shown experimentally in rats (Pozo et al. 1997) it also has a direct analgesic effect on joint nociceptors.

ROLE OF HYALURONIC ACID IN OSTEOARTHRITIS

Hyaluronic acid, one of the most important components of synovial fluid, is usually accepted as the protector of articular cartilage and soft tissue surfaces from injury during joint function. HA is an important, although minor component of the articular cartilage matrix, and it plays an important role in the aggregation of proteoglycans. Balazs et al. (1966) suggested that a 1–2 μ thick layer, which adheres to the articular cartilage surface, may contain HA, which may protect cartilage from wear and may also act as a shock absorber, protecting the cartilage from shock thrusts. Disturbances in the HA level in the synovial fluid may result in damage to the surface layer, and due to changes in the permeability proteins and other high molecular weight (HMW) substances may permeate into the cartilage matrix. Therefore, injection of HMW-HA may restore the damaged HA layer on the surface of articular cartilage, alleviating the arthritic condition and retarding the progress of the disease.

The overall role of the elastoviscous fluid, injected into the knee joint, has been deduced as to supplement and restore, the lubricating, protecting and shock absorbing properties of synovial fluid, which are compromized in osteoarthritis. After biomatrix, scientists introduced this system (in clinical medicine) known as viscosupplementation, it has been variously observed in relieving the pain and improving the mobility in osteoarthritic joint.

In the beginning, HA was extracted from bovine vitreous humor (had a MW of 15–20 × 10^4 and a protein content of ~10%), later Balazs et al. (1972) purified HA from human umbilical cord and rooster combs with a high MW (100–300 × 10^4), high viscosity and protein content of <1%. After obtaining good results with injecting the HA into arthritic and/or traumatic joint in the animals, intra-articular injection of HA was also observed to be effective in human being (Helfet 1974). At least there was no aggravation of the symptoms after HA injection.

In most of the cases, the effects of HA injection was seen in 2 days, however, the effects lasted variably from one week to 12 months (on an average 8 weeks).

Roman et al. (2000) opined that the best course of action appears to be one injection a week for 5 weeks, during which period the joint eliminates the excess of HA. Except some transient pain and local warmth lasting for 1–2 days, there was no adverse effect or any change in blood or urine. The immediate result was good-to-excellent in 41% of their patients. By 6 months, 75% of patients came down to fair relief or even no clinical response.

CORTICOSTEROIDS VERSUS HYALURONIC ACID

Like the effect of corticosteroids many patients begin to respond only after few HA injections but few may require even 8–10 injections to show the effect. However, the long-term effect may be satisfactory, especially in osteoarthritis. In animals (rabbits), repeated HA intra-articular injection was found to have a preventive effect (Namiki et al. 1975).

Lavelle et al. (2007) conducted a randomized, placebo-controlled study comparing >100 patients who were injected HA, corticosteroid (methylpredrisolone acetate) or isotonic saline, with the aid of ultrasound. Injections were given at the interval of 2 weeks—each patient recieving three injection. They observed significant improvement in patients recieving corticosteroid at 3 months as compared with those recieving isotonic saline, whereas the improvement in the patient, who were given HA, failed to reach the statistics significance. They did not find any significant difference betweeen the HA and corticosteroid at any point of observation.

Side Effects

Experimentally, even twice a week **HA intra-articular injection** for 6 months have been tolerated well in dogs without any side effect, however, in human beings 16 HA injections did not produce any adverse effects.

Intra-articular HA did not prove effective in osteoarthritic joints with effusion, probably because the scheduled effect of HA is nullified by the excessive joint fluid.

The efficacy and long-term benefit of intra-articular HA injection have not been yet clearly established. Further, the disadvantages of this treatment include the need for a minimum of initial three injections. Unlike corticosteroids, HA disappears from the joint cavity within a few days of intra-articular injection, hence long-lasting effect of HA cannot be explained by direct action of HA alone. Probably, it normalizes synovial fluid production and helps in the reconstruction of barrier protecting the synovial membrane and cartilage surface.

As corticosteroids do, HA does not have anti-inflammatory effects. Hence, if cocktail of HA and corticosteroids is injected, the overall results become superior than of either alone. Further, the dose of corticosteroids is reduced (half or even less) in future requirements to have some effect, thereby the possible adverse side effects of repeated corticosteroids injection can be avoided.

If compared for effects in osteoarthritic knee there is hardly any difference between patients treated with intra-articular injections of Hylan G-F_{20} (one course of 3 weekly injections) and those treated with corticosteroid (2–3 weekly injection) with respect to pain relief or functional improvement by 6–9 months follow-up.

A comparative experimental study with histopathologic evaluations have shown that corticosteroid is effective in the treatment of cartilage degeneration and inflammation early in the course of septic arthritis, whereas the therapeutic effect of hyaluronan is higher late in the course of the disease. However, further multicornered studies are required to draw proper conclusion (Karak et al. 2001).

As a practical approach, it appears that for a knee with effusion, corticosteroids injection should be considered after aspiration of effusion and for symptomatic dry knee HA injection may be more favourable choice.

Application of naturally found materials from biological sources and with possibilities to promote and accelerate bone and soft tissue healing. Platelet-rich plasma (PRP) is an orthobiologic and is becoming popular as an adjuvant treatment for musculoskeletal injuries. Other orthobiologics are bone marrow concentrates stem cells.

Platelet-rich plasma is potentially able to produce collagen, growth factor and probably also has the capacity to increase in number of available stem cells, which consequently enhances healing by delivering high concentration of alpha-granules containing biologically active moieties.

PLATELET-RICH PLASMA INJECTION

Since more than a decade, the role of PRP in enhancing the healing of injuries mainly of injuries mainly of tendons, ligaments, and even bones, and in managing the degenerative changes of joints involved in locomotor apparatus, is being discussed, albeit with no clear-cut outcome. The sports physicians, rheumatologists, radiologists and orthopedic surgeons have mainly used PRP.

Platelets (part of small solid components of blood-plasma) have important role in clotting the blood. The platelets also contain numerous proteins which have importance in healing the injuries and inflammation. The normally contained platelets in plasma are concentrated 5–10 times to prepare 'PRP'. For the process of concentration the blood is drawn from the patient, the platelets are separated from other blood cells and concentration of platelets is increased by centrifugation. Then the concentrated platelets are mixed with the remaining blood to prepare PRP. PRP can be given more precisely using ultrasound, which facilitates directly giving into the tissue.

***PRP has been used in the following conditions*:**

1. Chronic tendon injuries, like tennis elbow, knee and ankle sprains, chronic Achilles tendonitis (Gulefi et al. 2015), inflammation of patellar tendon (Jumpers knee), etc.
2. Acute sports injuries of muscles and pulled hamstrings; injuries of ligaments, e.g., in various sprains, torn ligaments.
3. PRP has been used during certain such as surgery of rotator cuff tendons, repair of torn anterior cruciate ligament, repair of completely torn heel cord—in this surgery PRP is prepared in a special way which it to be actually stitched into the torn tissue.
4. In certain swollen inflamed painful conditions of runners, tennis players and athletes, such as heel cord tendinosis, tennis elbow, a mixture of PRP and local anesthetics can be directly injected into the inflammed tissue. However, after an injection the area usually becomes more swollen and painful, albeit, the beneficial effects of injection appear after several weeks. In plantar fascitis PRP appears to be equally effective as the corticosteroid injection (Mahindra et al. 2016). However, in certain studies, PRP injection has been more effective in reducing pain and providing better functional results in comparatively long follow-up.
5. Several athletes have used PRP to return quickly for competition.
6. PRP has been used in degenerative arthritis of knee (Meheux et al. 2016) and ankle. In the ankle PRP injection was observed to be more effective than viscosupplementation or corticosteroid injection (Hue et al. 2016).

    The mode of working of PRP is not clearly understood. Increased content of protein growth factors has been given credit of potentially accelerating the healing process in the injured or diseased tissues of tendons, ligaments, muscles fascia and even for bone of foot).

7. The role of Photo-activated PRP (PA-PRP) has been found to be encouraging (such as in tendinitis, partial ligament tear). The PA-PRP is known to break the α-granules in the platelet which releases growth hormones. The growth hormone helps in repairing the partial tear of ligaments and also the resolution of inflammation.
8. In osteoarthritis (especially in bigger joints like knee) this biologically active substance—PRP injection into the joint, significantly reduces the pain and leads to better functional outcome compared to steroid injection (at least in early follow-ups.)
9. In a randomized control study comparing the efficacy of Triamcinolone injection versus PRP in Rotator Cuff Tendinopathy, initially Triamcinolone injection provided better results but on long-term follow-up the result of PRP was found to be superior (S Satish Kumar 2019).

Articular cartilage has limited intrinsic repairing capacity and cartilage defects can end in osteoarthritis. Therefore, procedures for stimulating cartilage repair are essential, even up to repair of full thickness cartilage defects. A recently developed technique is BioCartilage (Arthrex), a modified microfracture technique that uses micronized allogenic cartilage in combination with PRP to create a biochemically active scaffold populated by mesenchymal stem cells from the microfractured bed (Meretoja 2012). Several investigators have suggested a valid and additive effect of PRP of cartilage repair, in association with chondral matrix or osteochondral scaffolds.

In a comparative study regarding the use of corticosteroids and PRP injection for treating chronic planter fasciitis both appeared safe and effective treatment options. The corticosteroids showed better results- improvements as a whole—in the short-term whereas PRP showed better results in the long-term, however there appears no significant drop-of effect of corticosteroids even in long-term probably due to natural healing of the disease in the meantime (Shetty et al. 2019).

CHAPTER 7

Methodology

"Principles of scientific method: Simplicity, reliability, reproducibility, predictability."

—**SP**

CHAPTER OUTLINE

- Preparation
- Equipment
- Position of the patient
- Soap water cleaning of the part
- Certain considerations in relation to intra-articular and allied injections
- Sites for injection

PREPARATION

The part to be injected must be assessed thoroughly prior to injection, keeping in view:

1. Condition of skin at and around the point of prick.
2. Presence of infective disease in the joint or the environment (which is a contraindication).
3. Point of maximum tenderness (where relative and trial indications are laid down) which should be marked either with skin marker pencil or by nail edge (which does not disappear while preparing the skin for injection).
4. Accessibility of the joint, i.e., preferable route of infiltration. The part must be fully exposed (as far as practicable as if preparing for the orthopedic operation in that area).
5. In the patients who have effusion, it should be properly aspirated under strict aseptic care, before corticosteroid injection, and then there should be more improvement.

EQUIPMENT

- A sterile split towel **(Figure 7.1)**
- Two syringes, the pistons of which move smoothly
- A 20-gauge needle is most commonly used, although needle from 19 to 24 gauge may sometimes be required.

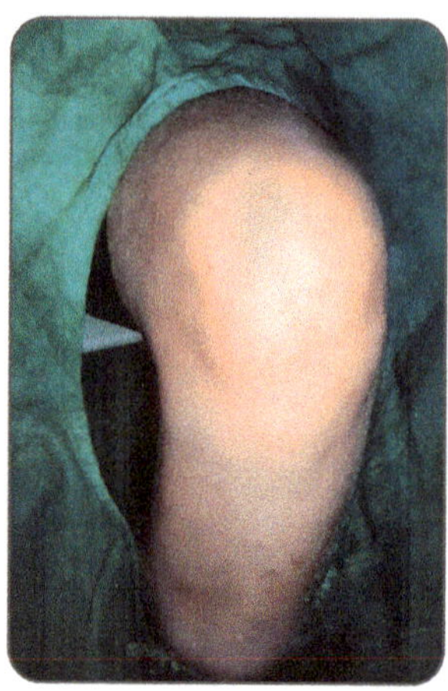

FIG. 7.1: Knee joint has been prepared for injection and sterilized split towel has been applied.

POSITION OF THE PATIENT

Many a times it becomes difficult to negotiate a needle through a joint space only for the faulty position of the patient. Hence, it is imperative that patient should be placed in a position which allows easy approach to the joint concerned (vide individual joint).

SOAP WATER CLEANING OF THE PART

This easy and always available procedure must be taken as mandatory. The fat solvent effect of the soap cleans the skin creases much more effectively, comparable to or even more than any other detergent or antiseptic solution. Areas well above and well below the site of prick should be thoroughly scrubbed, cleaned and washed out. Hair must be shaved from hairy areas.

CERTAIN CONSIDERATIONS IN RELATION TO INTRA-ARTICULAR AND ALLIED INJECTIONS

1. All intra-articular injections must be given in an operation theater environment in an aseptic surrounding. There is all danger of introducing infection through local injection therapy. Considering the corticosteroids, **NOT** only the millions of tiny microcrystals of corticosteroids physically protect the infective organisms from the access of the body defences, but the corticosteroids themselves suppress the local immune inflammatory response to infection. Hence, strict aseptic technique is mandatory.
2. The syringe, needle and other equipments must be thoroughly sterilized by autoclaving or prolonged boiling for minimum of 45 minutes or sterilized double layered packed disposable equipment should be used.

3. The joint along with wide areas in the surroundings must be thoroughly cleaned by repeated soap water/detergents and/or chlorhexidine gluconate-cetrimide and rectified spirit and/or microbicidal solutions (e.g., povidone-iodine available as Betadine) or allied antiseptics.
4. The stopper of corticosteroid/methyl prednisolone acetate or hydrocortisone acetate and local anesthetic vials must be thoroughly cleaned by above lotions.
5. The surgeon must scrub thoroughly and use a pair of sterilized gloves.
6. After antiseptic procedures, as far as possible, always avoid touching the part to be injected. However, if it is essential to localize the point of prick, an antiseptic swab mopping must precede the needle prick.
7. It is beneficial to use a sharp, fine needle (20–24 gauges). Though hydrocortisone acetate is a suspension, we had not a single occasion to repent for not using the wide-bore needle for intra-articular injection. The injection remains almost painless.

   Thoroughly sterilized double-layered packed disposable syringes, needles and gloves should be used.
8. A controlled sharp quick push through the joint space gives very little trouble to the patient. Whatever possible, the joint fluid should be aspirated, inspected and sent for culture. If the fluid is opaque or other than the normal synovial fluid look, corticosteroid should not be injected, rather inject some antibiotics if there is any doubt of any infection (e.g., kanamycin).
9. Always avoid touching the bone or cartilage surface by the needle-end. Somehow or other, it hurts the patient instantaneously and pain persists for varying periods, sometimes even days together. In certain cases, effusion and swelling develop. However, it settles with assurances, ice-cold compress, rest to the part and analgesic. Theoretical risks always exist causing damage to articular cartilage by the sharp needle point and also by the chemical activity of the corticosteroids which is likely to soften the articular cartilage predisposing to tear.
10. Local anesthetic is not necessary if proper techniques are applied. However, when it is essential, keep the needle in situ after injecting local anesthetic, detach the syringe to load the corticosteroid or cocktail; do not leave but the end of the needle open to exterior; rather, put a sterilized small cotton wool over the needle-end to avoid contamination with the environmental air.

    One dilemma in using the local anesthetic may disappoint the patient against which they should be warned. With local anesthetics the patient may feel instant relief, but pain returns after the anesthetics effect wears off.
11. It has been seen that in an over-enthusiastic attempt to inject the last droplet of drug, some air is pushed into. It must be avoided, at least it is going to increase the bulk in the joint space besides potentially carrying the possibility of infection (unless it is done in the modern sterile-air operation theater environment).

12. After taking out the needle, few droplets/drops of blood may come out. A gentle, local to-and-fro massage automatically seals the passage. However, it is always better to seal the prick with tincture of benzoin or povidine-iodine. Be cautious where you are injecting in a joint where someone else has previously given an injection and when the technique might not have been that meticulous as should be. In such cases, send the adequate fluid for culture.
13. Following injection of corticosteroid ask the patient to gently move the joint or part as far as practicable or you passively move it to the possible range. This helps in dispersal of the injected material. If needed the joint should be moved few times passively.
14. Patient must not be allowed to be up and about immediately after the prick. There can be psychological fear, vasovagal attack and allergic reactions to lidocaine hydrochloride or other materials used.
15. The patient should be restrained from immediate vigorous use of the limb or exercises. About 24 hours abstinence from unnecessary vigorous activities or exercises or walking (in case of lower limb) provides comfort to the patient in subsequent activities or physiotherapy. This helps by providing a time for biological adaptation. In any case, the patient should be firmly warned not to apply untoward stress on the joint injected.
16. More than one joint can be injected at a time but let it be not more than four joints in one sitting, e.g., in rheumatoid arthritis. After all we are dealing with living human creatures and the patient may not be able to use his several joints for variable period. As such even 125 mg of hydrocortisone acetate or more (and comparable amount of other corticosteroids) can be used at a time without any complication.
17. If there is pain after intra-articular injections, initially ice pack application helps in allaying pain. After 12–16 hours, hot moist fomentation may be useful. It helps in allaying the associated inflammatory process, if any. Further, counter-irritant effect of heat allays the pain following the prick.
18. There is hardly any systemic effect of local corticosteroid injection, however, rarely improvements occur in other (than one injected) joints, which may be due to the systemic effects of the injected corticosteroids ultimately entering the blood stream with the same explanation. There may be very rare risk of adrenal cortical suppression after repeated corticosteroid injections and it may produce theoretical hazards of inadequate adrenal cortical response to the stresses.
19. One should always be apprehensive of aggravating the infection after injecting into an already infected joint. However, sometimes the patients of chronic arthritis with damaged joints (e.g., rheumatoid arthritis) already treated by oral corticosteroids do not manifest the systemic constitutional features of infection, and in such cases it is difficult to clinically diagnose the pyogenic infection of the joint and one may inject the corticosteroids in such infected joints. However, it is always safe to aspirate the fluid and send for culture before injection therapy.

Sometimes after local injection, the pain increases with features of inflammation, giving rise to worries about iatrogenic infection. However, microcrystalline suspensions of corticosteroids may induce temporary crystal synovitis like gout producing the inflammatory features. This should be managed by rest, NSAID, cold compress, and reassurance along with prophylactic antibiotics.

20. Like **CompuMed (computer controlled local anesthetic delivery system**—a revolution, any system that allows to easily deliver virtually painfree injections of local anesthetic) corticosteroid can also be given which will have much patient's acceptability. The **CompuMed system** provides microprocessor control for more precise and predictable drug delivery.

SITES FOR INJECTION

In orthopedic practice, corticosteroids have been used for:

- Intra-articular
- Periarticular local infiltration
- Intratendinous—very cautiously limited prick, since it may predispose to rupture of the tendon
- Peritendinous
- Intranodular
- Perinodular injection
- Intraganglionic and periganglionic (When ganglion is in relation to the tendinous stretch)
- Intraneural—e.g., in **Hansen's neuritis** into peripheral nerves (e.g., ulnar, lateral popliteal nerves, etc.)
- Perineural
- Epidural injection.

In most of the joints, intra-articular injections are needed, but few joints suffering from periarticular adhesive capsulitis lesions (e.g., shoulder joint) do require periarticular infiltration. Carette et al. (2003) have reported significant improvement in frozen shoulder with corticosteroid injections with exercises compared to by exercises alone. Eustace et al. (1997) concluded from their studies that about 68% of the shoulder injections, given even by experts with radiological guidance failed to enter into the glenohumeral joint.

In selecting the site of injection for a joint following points must be considered:

1. Approach should be direct straight (not in curved/or circuitous route) into the joint.
2. Prick must avoid major blood vessels and nerves.
3. As far as possible, joint-line should be first located.

If blood uniformly mixed with joint fluid is aspirated, suspect trauma (hemarthrosis—blood appears more thicker and veinous and with sparkling fat globules) or bleeding disease. In such situation, hemarthrosis should be aspirated, and some prophylactic antibiotic may be injected but corticosteroids should not be injected.

Possibility of damage to articular cartilage by the sharp point of needle always exists, which must be avoided as far as possible. It is liable to predispose softening of the cartilage (further accentuated by the chemical activities of the injected corticosteroids).

After corticosteroid injection there is the possibility of **aseptic necrosis of the joint surface** due to infarction of the subchondral bone. However, such lesions may exist prior to injection as well, e.g., in hips, knees, ankles, especially in severe rheumatoid arthritis, and cartilage breakdown after local corticosteroid injection in these joints may be just coincidental.

Sometimes following the injections of long-acting corticosteroids in superficial joints (e.g., knee, PIP or DIP joints) some of the injected material may leak out through the injection tract and cause some discoloration (e.g., whitish patch) and atrophy of overlying skin with increased transparency. However, the whitish patch disappears in due course. The patient must be informed (cautioned) about this possibility prior to giving injection.

CHAPTER 8

Shoulder Joint

"A creative man is motivated by the desire to achieve,
NOT by the desire to beat others."

—Ayn Rand

CHAPTER OUTLINE

- Anterior approach
- Posterior approach
- Periarthritic infiltration
- Anterolateral approach

In all approaches the point of prick should be ascertained and marked by skin pencil or nail edge before preparing the part antiseptically. One of the main concerns with shoulder injections is the delivering of steroids into the glenohumeral joint. In good number of cases injections given by experts, even with radiological guidance, fail to enter into the glenohumeral joint. Further, the efficacy of corticosteroids intra-articular injections in treating frozen shoulder is still questionable. However, when combined with physiotherapy, it usually reduces pain and disability.

ANTERIOR APPROACH

The patient lies supine with arm by the side of chest and shoulder girdle well-supported on the sandbag. Feel the tip of the coracoid process, just outside it, a narrow depression can be felt, extending more downwards than upwards. The fingertip can be hardly insinuated in it. Mark it by skin pencil or nail edge before preparing it antiseptically. In the depression, the needle should be pushed posteriorly with slight outward and downward inclination. Usually, no resistance is felt and needle may be pushed up to hilt **(Figure 8.1)**.

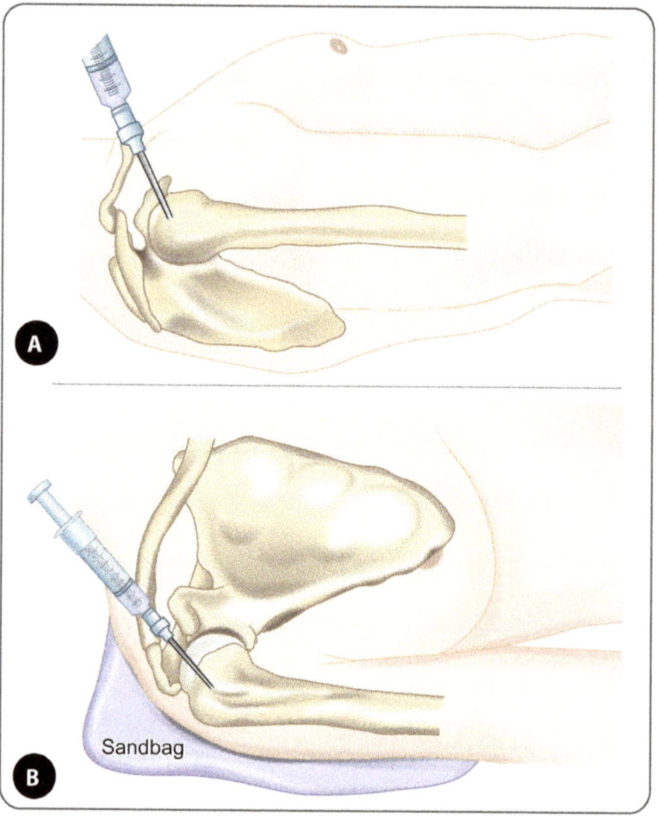

FIGS. 8.1A AND B: Shoulder joint (anterior approach). Viewed from side (A); from above (B).

POSTERIOR APPROACH

This approach is suitable for periarthritic infiltration. However, it can also be used for injecting into the joint. Patient lies by the side with the joint to be injected above. Posterior acromion angle is felt. Just lateral to and behind it, a finger-tip can be insinuated into a depression. Mark it before preparing for injection. A needle may be introduced through it, anteriorly with very little (about 15°) downward inclination **(Figure 8.2)**.

Periarthritic local infiltration is significantly effective in pain control, early mobilization, and recovery of functions with the lesser consumption of analgesics postoperatively. On the whole it is more effective with greater patient's satisfaction and even lesser consumption of analgesics postoperatively. On the whole it is more effective with patient's satisfaction even when compared to the use of buprenorphine transdermal patch.

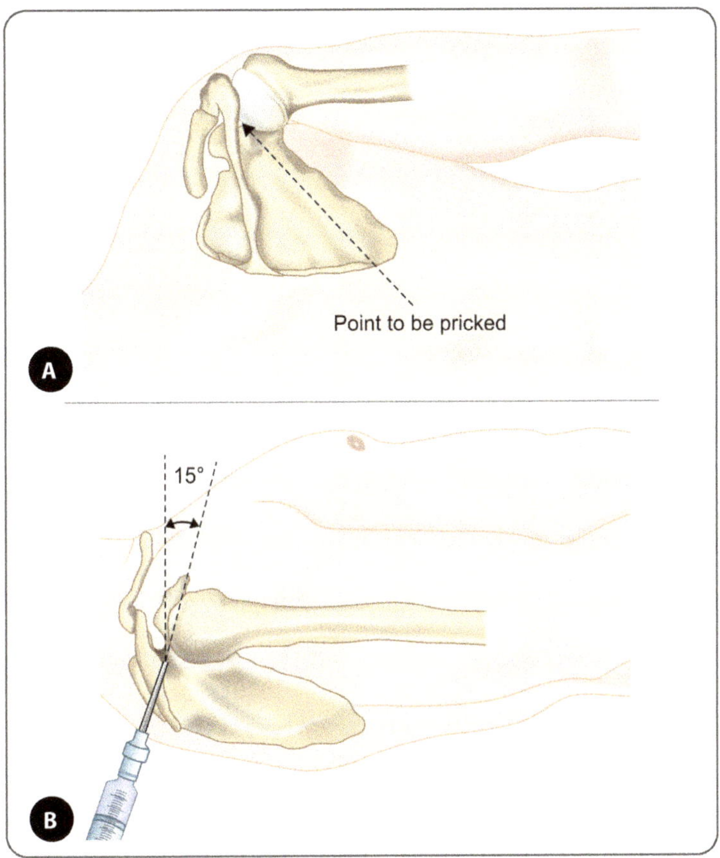

FIGS. 8.2A AND B: Shoulder joint (posterior approach). Viewed from back (A); from above (B).

PERIARTHRITIC INFILTRATION

The patient lies on his side with the arm to be injected resting on the side of chest. Posterior acromion angle is felt. Just lateral and behind it, finger-tip can be insinuated into a depression. Through it, a needle is pushed anteriorly with 15-20 degrees downwards and outwards inclination **(Figure 8.3)**. Pricking up to the hilt of the needle is without any resistance. As the drug is injected, one may see slight puffing just anteriorly. This is due to pouching out of subacromion bursa.

Periarthritic infiltration may be done in sitting posture also, however, lying down position should be preferred. Patient sits on a stool against the back of the upright of a chair, kept infront of him/her. The lower portion of both forearms rest on the arms of the chair from behind. Automatically, the arms lie in slight flexion, abduction and internal rotation position.

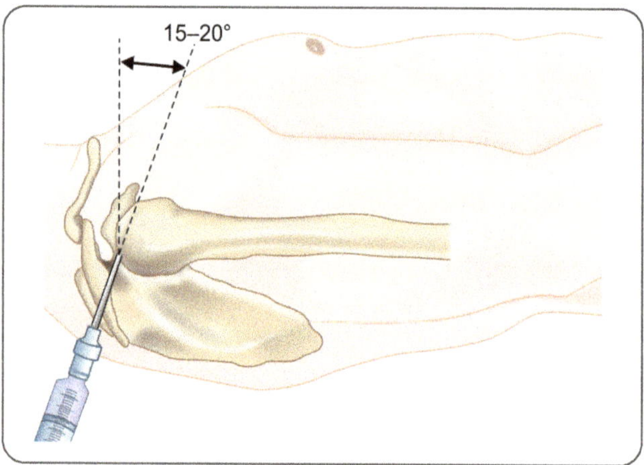

FIG. 8.3: Shoulder joint—approach for periarthritic infiltration.

Feel the posterior angle of acromion. Just below and outside it, a sharp depression is felt. Push the needle forward with a slight medial and downward inclination **(Figure 8.3)**.

ANTEROLATERAL APPROACH

In bicipital tenosynovitis, corticosteroid infiltration can be done into the sheath of biceps tendon as well as in bicipital groove. The patient lies supine with a sandbag beneath the shoulder. The most tender point is sought on the anterolateral slope of the shoulder top. Occasionally a thickened, tender band can be rolled under the finger **(Figure 8.4)**.

The needle should be pushed from below upwards with an inclination backwards and laterally for infiltration into the sheath **(Figure 8.5)**. As the sheath is entered into, one can see and test, to-and-fro movements of the detached needle with contraction and relaxation of biceps tendon. After injecting into the sheath the needle can be pushed further backwards to enter into the bicipital groove, a bony resistance is felt as the floor of bicipital groove is reached. The tendon should not be infiltrated into, only it should be bathed from all around.

Intra-articular distention in the management of capsulitis of the shoulder (6 mL 0.25% bupivacaine and 3 mL of air) has been found to be superior to the intra-articular injection of steroid alone (40 mg triamcinolone acetonide in 1 mL). However, more improvement was observed when steroid and distension were combined, with distension probably acting synergistically (Jacobs LGH et al. 1991). Posterior route to glenohumeral joint should be employed for injection and distension.

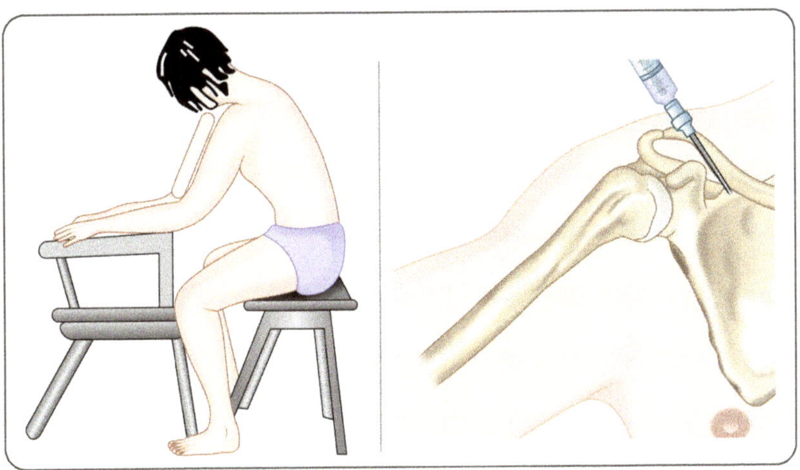

FIG. 8.4: Shoulder joint—approach in sitting position.

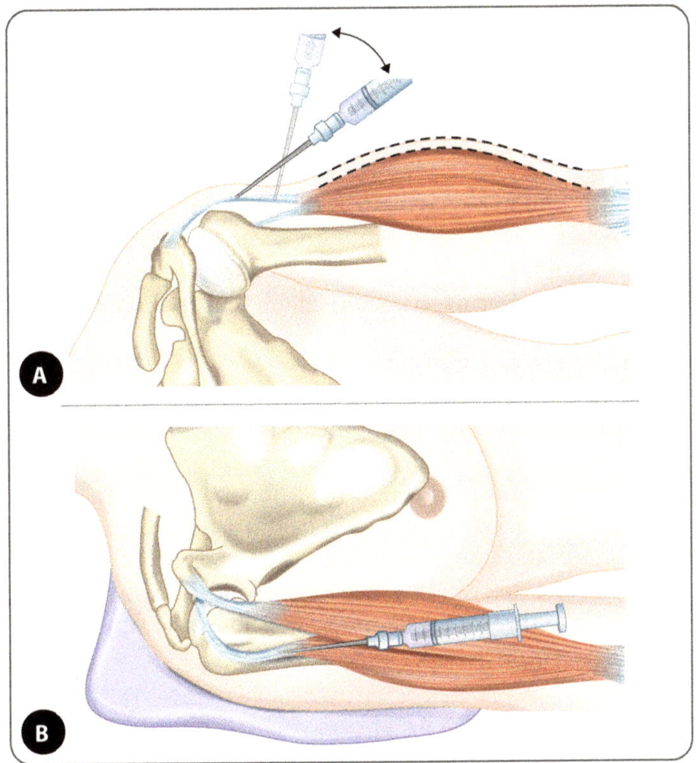

FIGS. 8.5A AND B: Infiltration for bicipital tenosynovitis. Viewed from side (A); from above (B).

CHAPTER 9

Elbow Joint

"Remain cool to reach your goal safe and fast."

—PP Wangchuk

CHAPTER OUTLINE

- Lateral approach
- Posterior approach
- Lateral epicondylitis (extra-articular tennis elbow)
- Olecranon bursitis
- Medial epicondylitis (golfer's elbow, pitcher's elbow, little league elbow syndrome)

Elbow is a composite joint having ulnohumeral, radiohumeral and radio-ulnar components. These have continuous and communicating synovial reflections. Therefore, if the drug is injected into one component, it easily spreads into other compartments, unless there is intra-articular adhesions.

LATERAL APPROACH

Lateral approach is through radiohumeral compartment. The patient lies supine. The arm is kept in slight internal rotation at shoulder. The elbow is flexed 30–40° from zero extension, with forearm in midprone position. A transverse slit can be felt at the posterolateral aspect just below the lateral epicondylar region. Further confirmation can be done by rotating the forearm in which radial head is felt rotating just beneath the slit. The needle is pushed into the slit having a direction anteriorly with about 20° upward inclination **(Figure 9.1)**.

POSTERIOR APPROACH

The patient lies on the side with the affected limb above. Elbow is flexed about 45° with forearm in midprone position. The olecranon tip stands prominent. On either side of the olecranon process a vertical slit can be felt. At a convenient point along the slit, a needle can be pushed on either side of the olecranon, having a direction downwards and toward mid-line **(Figure 9.2)**.

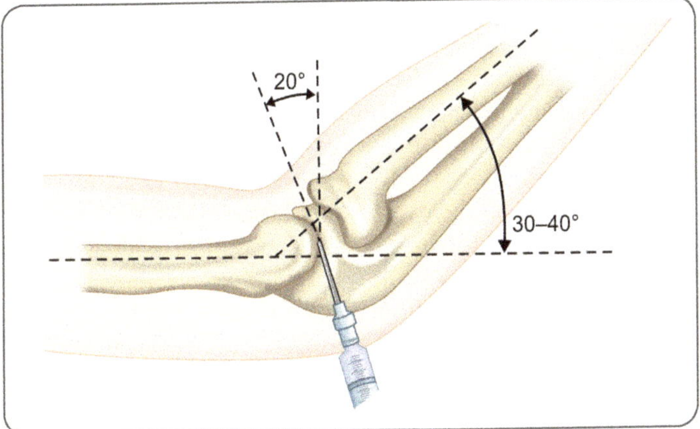

FIG. 9.1: Elbow joint—lateral approach.

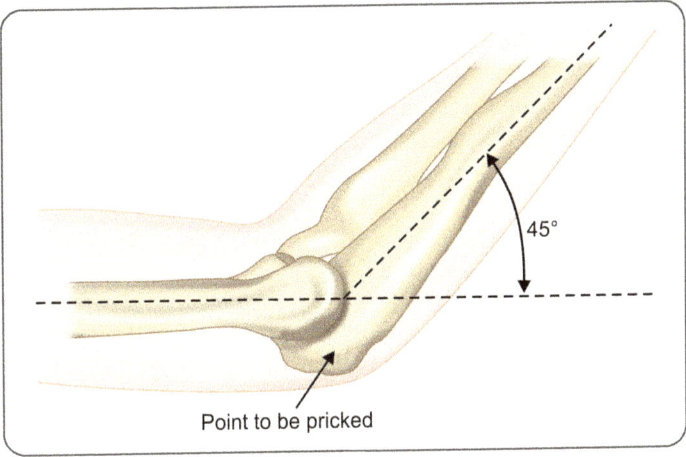

FIG. 9.2: Elbow joint—posterior approach.

LATERAL EPICONDYLITIS (EXTRA-ARTICULAR TENNIS ELBOW)

Lateral epicondylitis (tennis elbow) has been recognized for over 100 years. It is an enthesopathy of the common extensors origin in the lateral epicondylar region, however, its pathogenesis is not clear. It has been also recognized as an overuse syndrome (repetitive stress disorder) due to repetitive tension overloading of the wrist extensor origin at the lateral epicondylar region.

First clinical description of lateral epicondylitis was given by Runge in 1873. More than 40 different types of treatment have been used alone or in combinations, e.g., anti-inflammatory drugs, steroids, physiotherapy techniques, cast immobilization, orthosis, surgery and less conventional methods such as radiotherapy, acupuncture and vitamins (Labelle et al.

1992). Recently, **extracorporeal shock-wave therapy (ESWT)** has been used in tennis elbow. The **mobile lithotripter** (2,000 shock waves at 2.5 bars of air pressure with a frequency of 8–10 Hz)—a total of three sittings at an interval of 2 weeks, each lasting for 3–4 minutes is an effective way of treating tennis elbow and plantar fascitis but it requires, further trials for authentication. However, it is much costly as compared to corticosteroids injection (100 times) and also less effective. By and large injection of corticosteroids along with hyaluronidase and local anesthetic is more effective treatment of tennis elbow.

In the elbow region, it is the commonest indication. Infiltration in such cases is done in and around the origin of common extensors from anteroinferior aspect of lateral epicondylar region. The patient lies supine. The elbow is kept in 45° flexion in midprone position. The anteroinferior part of lateral epicondylar region is easily felt. Palpate over the bony region and its adjoining area for locating the maximum tenderness. The most tender point is directly injected pushing the needle almost up to subperiosteal region. The adjoining areas should also be infiltrated **(Figure 9.3)**. It is better to manipulate at the elbow in the same sitting. Hold the hand of the patient in your right hand in the handshake position. Support the elbow from behind by your left hand. While gently rotating the forearm and flexing/extending at elbow, give a sudden jerky extension to the elbow. You may hear a mild click. Quite often it gives good relief, probably by virtue of breaking the fibrotic adhesions.

OLECRANON BURSITIS

Olecranon bursitis **(Figure 9.4)** is the inflammation of the bursa overlying the olecranon process caused by repetitive or even acute trauma. It presents as a more or less round tense, fluctuant (may not be demonstrable), tender

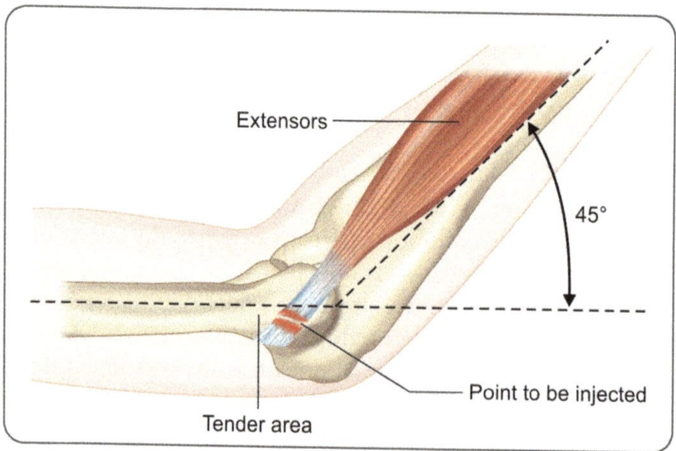

FIG. 9.3: Elbow joint—approach of extra-articular tennis elbow.

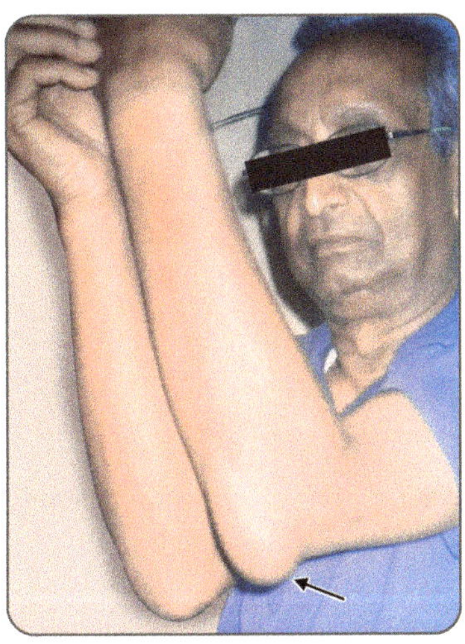

FIG. 9.4: Olecranon bursitis on left elbow.

swelling. It should be aspirated from the nondependent side (to avoid leakage after withdrawing the needle). Usually no local anesthetic is required. The aspiration needle is advanced while maintaining negative pressure in the syringe. When the fluid starts flowing in the syringe, the needle is no longer advanced further. If the fluid is clear, the needle should be left in situ and other syringe containing the steroid is changed to inject it slowly after the aspirate stopped flowing. It may prevent recurrence. The fluid should be sent for examination and culture, especially if the fluid is not clear.

MEDIAL EPICONDYLITIS (GOLFER'S ELBOW, PITCHER'S ELBOW, LITTLE LEAGUE ELBOW SYNDROME)

It is an overuse syndrome, common in young persons and is caused by chronic tension stress injuries, repetitive tension overloading of the flexor-pronator muscles at or near its origin from the medial epicondyle.

When the problem does not improve with noninvasive methods (as noted in lateral epicondylitis) local infiltration of the corticosteroid cocktail should be done in the flexor-pronator muscles origin complex just at and near the medial epicondyle.

Method

Patient lies supine with shoulder abducted (by 90°), elbow flexed by 40° and forearm supinated. The medial epicondyle is palpated and maximum tender point is spotted and marked by skin pencil or nail edge. After preparing the skin antiseptically, the needle is pushed from just below the medial epicondylar tip in the upward and anterior direction. Just before reaching the bone, the medicine is pushed infiltrating the zone.

CHAPTER 10

Wrist Joint

"Calmness of mind is one of the beautiful jewels of wisdom."

—James Allen

CHAPTER OUTLINE

- Approaches for wrist joint
- De Quervain's disease
- Injection approaches for metacarpophalangeal joints and interphalangeal joints
- Trigger thumb/finger

For all practical purposes, wrist joint behaves as a composite joint, consisting of radiocarpal joint, intercarpal joints and inferior radioulnar joint. These have intercommunicating synovial reflections. But, intercarpal joints being very snugly spaced, drugs pushed into these joints can hardly reach the inferior radioulnar joint. In most of the cases requiring corticosteroid injection, the inferior radioulnar joint is at fault, especially after trauma in and around the wrist joint.

APPROACHES FOR WRIST JOINT

In post-traumatic conditions (of which the most common is malunited **Colles fracture**) pressure at the tip of the ulnar styloid process initiates pain and is most tender. It is either due to fibrous healing of the avulsed ulnar styloid process, or mild persistent subluxation of inferior radioulnar joint, or inferior radioulnar traumatic synovitis or arthritis. In such conditions, local infiltration beneath and around the tip of ulnar styloid process can be done directly. For injecting into the wrist joint and/or into the inferior radioulnar joint following methods may be followed:

a. The patient lies supine and keeps the wrist in prone position. Feel the ulnar styloid process. Just beneath and behind it there is a depression. Through it push the needle radialwards with about 20° of upward and foreward inclination **(Figure 10.1)**.

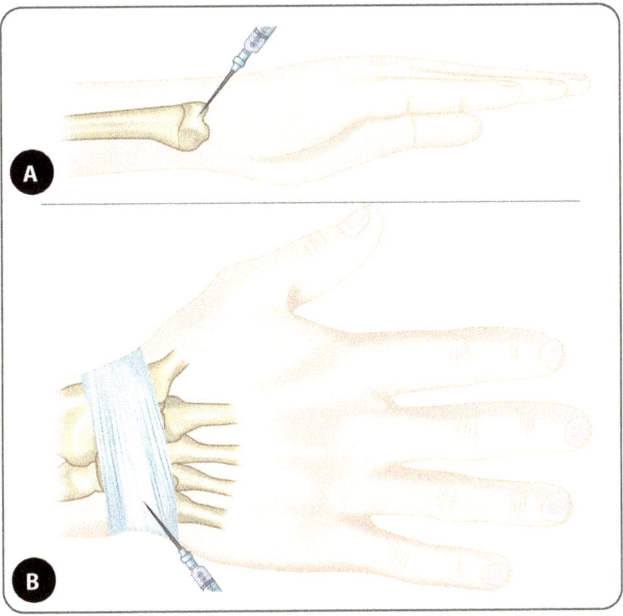

FIGS. 10.1A AND B: Wrist joint—approach from ulnar side. Lateral view (A); Dorsal view (B).

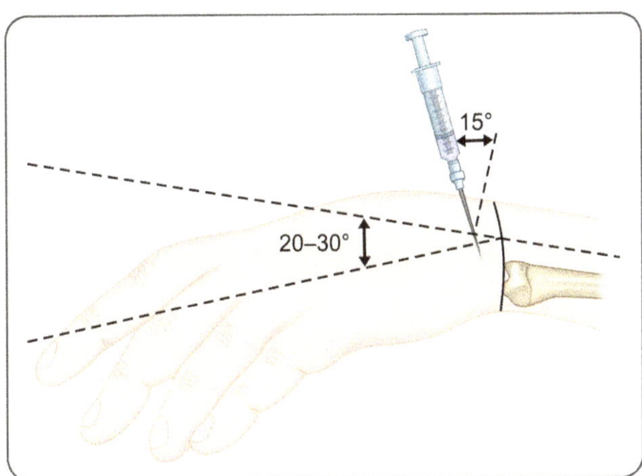

FIG. 10.2: Wrist joint—approach from dorsum.

b. In fully prone position of the hand, wrist is flexed to about 20-30°. About 0.5 cm below the midinterstyloid line, an yield or depression can be felt on the dorsum of wrist. The needle can be pushed through the gap almost anteriorly with 15° upward inclination **(Figure 10.2)**.

DE QUERVAIN'S DISEASE

In the wrist region, perhaps, the most common use of corticosteroid injection is in the De Quervain's disease (stenosing tenosynovitis of the abductor pollicis longus and extensor pollicis brevis tendon) and ganglion. The firm and tendor swelling in this disease is obvious above the radial styloid process **(Figure 10.3)**.

Method

The patient lies supine. In mid-prone position of the hand, the needle is pushed, starting about 1 cm above the styloid process, below upwards in the direction of abductor pollicis longus tendon. When the sheath is supposed to be entered into, the needle should be disconnected from the syringe and the patient is asked to abduct and extend the thumb repeatedly. With each movement the needle moves to-and-fro with playing of the tendon. This should be tested before injecting the drug, since it ensures delivery of drug at proper site.

Another common indication around the wrist is for a ganglion, **(Figures 10.4 and 10.5)**. Ganglion must be pitched and injected into directly. For the ganglion associated with any tendon, to-and-fro movements of the needle after penetrating the sheath of that tendon should be tested with the movement of that particular tendon. The ganglion should be made prominent by contracting the particular tendon before injecting into it. If it lies deep to the tendon, it will not become prominent, but will be fixed with contraction of

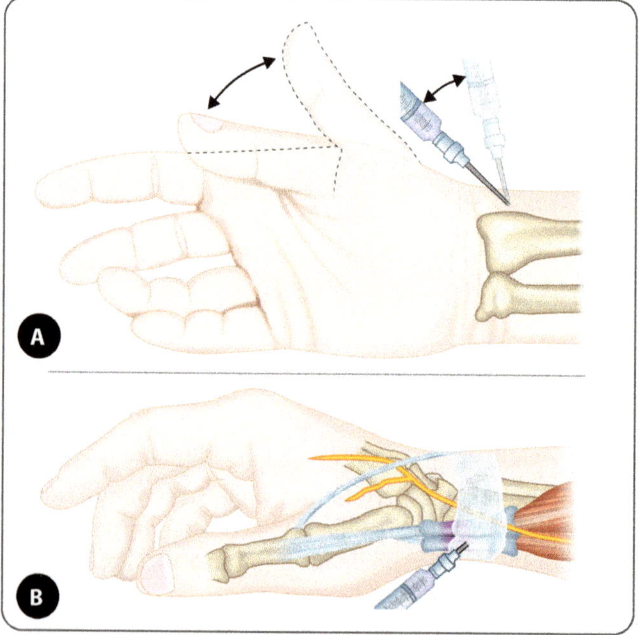

FIGS. 10.3A AND B: Approach for De Quervain's disease. Viewed from side (A); Needle into tendon sheath (B).

the tendon, which will facilitate the injection. Ganglion communicating with the wrist or carpal joints diminish in size or disappear following dorsiflexion of the wrist joint. Hence, it should be made prominent by palmar-flexing the wrist or planer-flexing the ankle in case of ganglion of the foot before injection **(Figures 10.3C and 10.4)**.

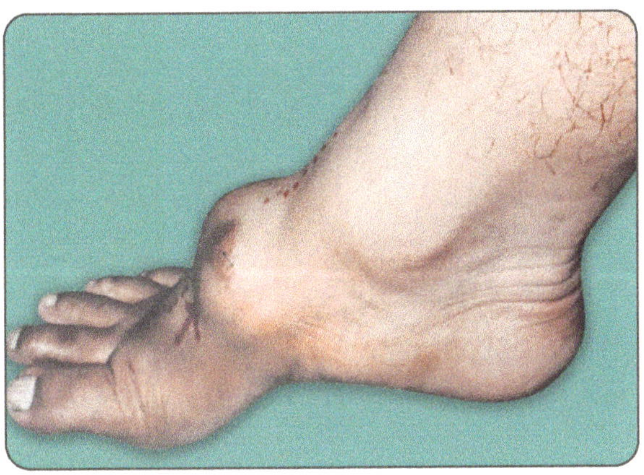

FIG. 10.3C: Note that when the person plantar flexes the foot the ganglion goes down and becomes more prominent.

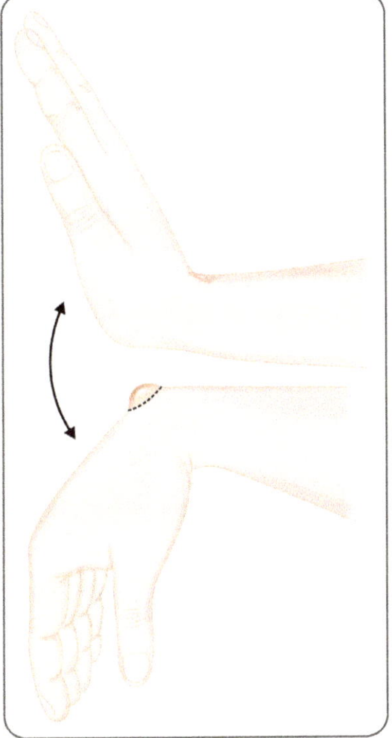

FIG. 10.4: Test showing intra-articular ganglion.

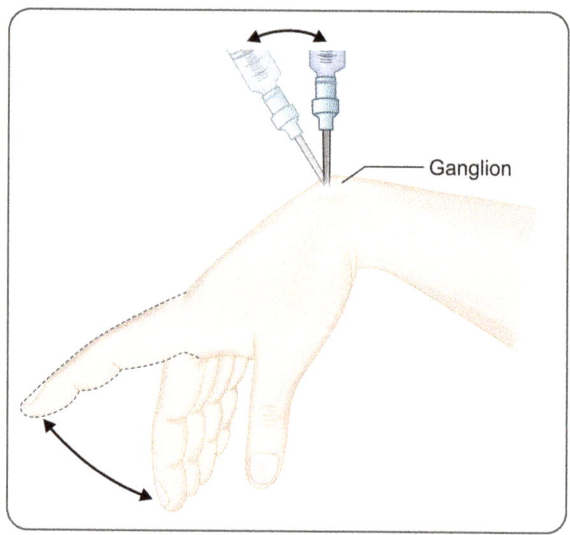

FIG. 10.5: Injection into ganglion of extensor tendon of index finger.

Prominent ganglion should be aspirated by a comparatively wide bore (No. 18G) needle. The aspirated material is clear jelly-like. One to three pricks into the ganglion from different angles facilitate the aspiration. Then, the ganglion should be squeezed and pressed from different visible directions. The size and prominence of ganglion become obviously smaller. Then, the corticosteroid mixed with hyaluronidase should be injected into the ganglion. The recurrence rate after the above procedure is markedly reduced. Usually, two to three injections are required at the interval of 2–3 weeks. Recurrence of ganglion is not uncommon at months/even years interval. Operation—excision of ganglion should be avoided as far as possible, since, it also does not guarantee against recurrence and it also produces, (ugly) scar on the visible aspect which looks more ugly than ganglion itself.

By the use of hyaluronidase the results of ganglion aspiration can be improved. The good effect has also been observed in treating **De Quervain's disease**.

INJECTION APPROACHES FOR METACARPOPHALANGEAL JOINTS AND INTERPHALANGEAL JOINTS

Flexing the particular joint by about 45°, a narrow transverse slit can be felt by gentle palpation, especially by the nail edge. Confirm it by repeatedly flexing and extending the joint. The fine needle can be pushed into the joint through the slit. Periarticular infiltration should also be done, if there is suspicion of periarticular adhesions **(Figure 10.6)**.

The metacarpophalangeal and interphalangeal joints can also be approached through the slit, felt on either side of joint, in about 45° flexed position of that particular joint **(Figure 10.7)**.

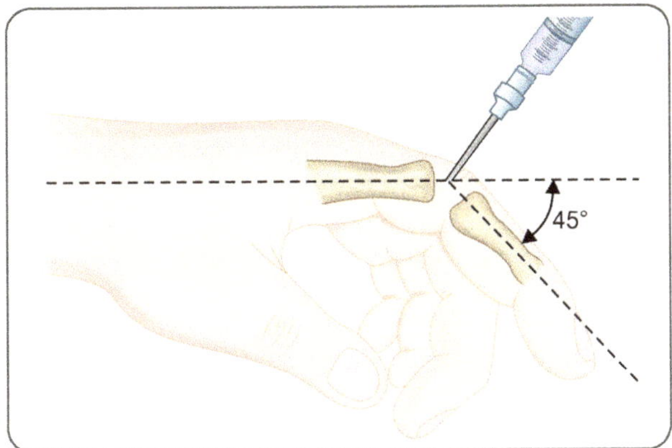

FIG. 10.6: Approach to interphalangeal joint from dorsum.

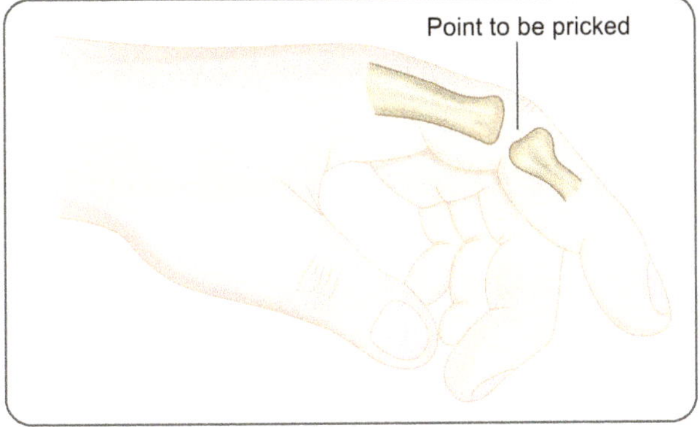

FIG. 10.7: Approach to interphalangeal joint from side.

TRIGGER THUMB/FINGER (FIGURE 10.8)

A common indication of corticosteroid injection in thumb or finger is trigger-thumb and trigger-finger. In this condition, the patient complains of temporary locking of the thumb or finger in the flexed position, to a varying extent. The finger can be extended by using more power for extension and jerky release is felt. One can palpate the firm tender nodule in the course of the concerned tendon, usually at the root of thumb on the palmar aspect, and along the lines of ring and middle fingers, distal to the distal palmar crease. These nodules are due to localized circumferential fibrosis in the tendon-sheath. Usually, injection is most effective within 3–4 weeks of the onset of pain and early triggering of the finger. As the nodule gets firmer, infiltrating of corticosteroids may be effective in reducing the pain to varying extent, but nodule persists and pain usually recurs. In such cases surgical slitting-open of the tendon-sheath in the nodular region gives almost cure.

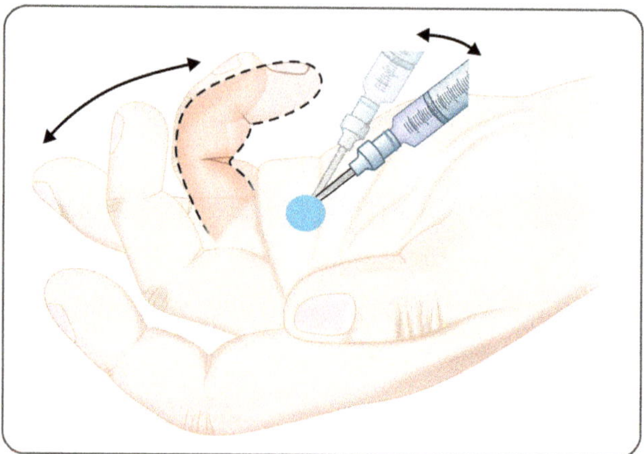

FIG. 10.8: Approach for trigger ring finger.

Method

By a direct approach just proximal or distal to the nodule, the local anesthetic may be infiltrated by the needle. The nodule is pithed and the tendon-sheath is entered into. A to and fro movements of needle is tested with excursion of that particular tendon before injecting the drug **(Figure 10.8)**.

CHAPTER 11

Hip Joint

"Failure is not falling down, but refusing to get up."

—A Chinese Proverb

CHAPTER OUTLINE

- Anterior approach
- Lateral approach

The degenerative changes in the hip joints, either primary or secondary to various conditions, are quite common. The corticosteroid injection is effective in degenerative arthrosis of the hip joint. Because of the difficult access to the hip joint proper, especially in nondistended capsule, intra-articular injection of corticosteroids could not be that popular. However, nowadays under the image guidance of ultrasound or fluoroscopy (which are proving to be a valuable tool to help access the difficult joints like hip and spinal joints) the hip joint can be more frequently injected. The approaches for injecting into the hip joint can be anterior or posterolateral.

ANTERIOR APPROACH (FIGURE 11.1)

The patient lies supine. Feel the femoral pulsation just below and outside the mid-inguinal point. About a finger-breadth out to it, will be the suitable point to approach the hip joint, i.e., about 2–3 cm below the anterior superior iliac spine and 2–3 cm lateral to the femoral pulse. Push the needle posteriorly with an inclination downwards and medially at an angle of about 60° with the skin through the hip capsule until bone is reached. Then the tip of needle is slightly withdrawn. In lucky situation, a drop or two of synovial fluid can be aspirated, which will confirm the penetration into the joint capsule. Under image intensifier, however, the needle can be manipulated comparatively easily into the hip joint. Even if bigger dose of corticosteroid is injected, the ball and socket joint of such a big dimension perhaps hurdles in spreading the drug over the inflamed synovial reflections of the joint.

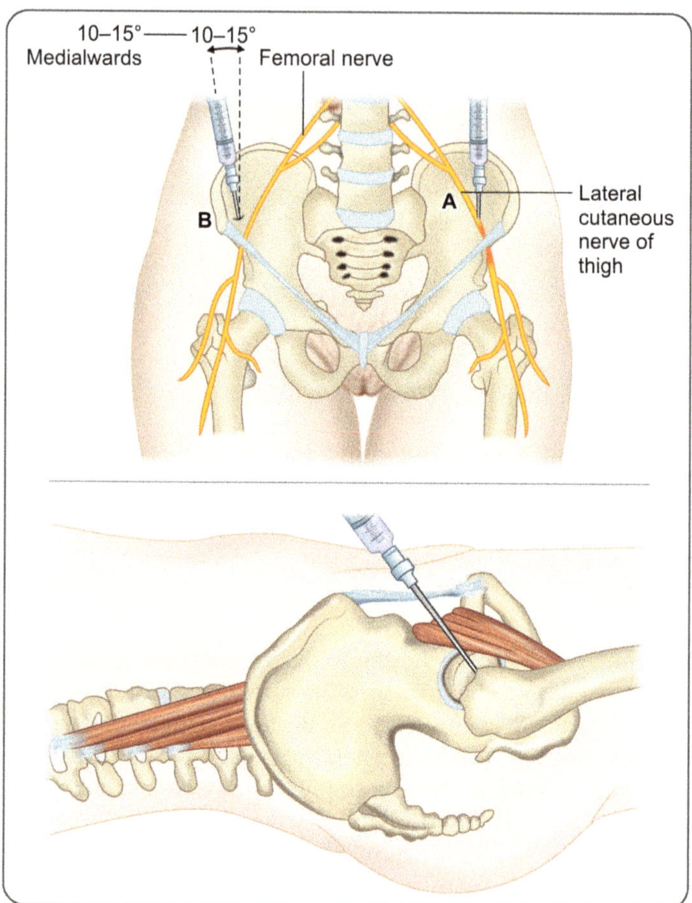

FIG. 11.1: Above (right side)—anterior approach to hip joint; (left side)—approach for meralgia paresthetica. Below—anterior approach to hip joint: Viewed from side.

LATERAL APPROACH (FIGURE 11.2)

It is also a difficult approach, however with a slender long needle, hip can be penetrated into. In this approach, there is advantage that the needle follow the bone to the hip joint. The patient lies in lateral position with the joint to be injected kept above. The needle is inserted just anterior to the greater trochanter in a sagittal direction pointing toward the mid-inguinal point. The needle tip slides anterior to the periosteum of the femoral neck and enters the hip joint space anteriorly.

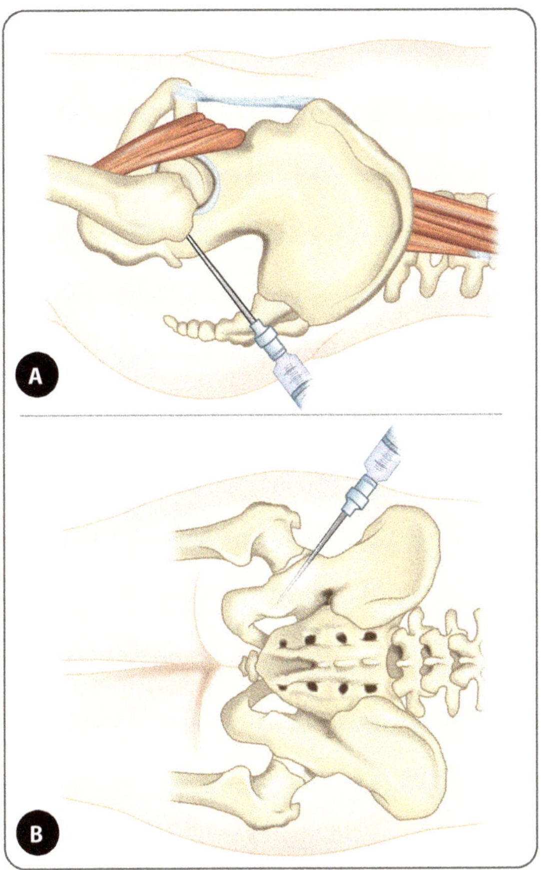

FIGS. 11.2A AND B: Posterolateral approach. Viewed from above (A); from back (B).

Meralgia Paresthetica

The corticosteroid injection is also given for **meralgia paresthetica** (entrapment of lateral cutaneous nerve of thigh under the outer end of inguinal ligament). The injection should be in cocktail of corticosteroid, hyaluronidase and lignocaine. The injection may be effective when given in early stage. Later on surgery seems to be inevitable, even though the result may not be uniformly good.

Method (Figure 11.1)

The patient lies supine. Select a point about a finger breadth medial to anterior superior iliac spine. Push the needle at this point with an inclination down to about subcutaneous depth. Slowly infiltrate corticosteroid cocktail vertically downwards in the area of about 3 cm at the depth of about 1 cm.

CHAPTER 12

Knee Joint

"Continuous effort—not strength or intelligence is the key to unlocking our potential."

—Winston Churchill

CHAPTER OUTLINE

- Why intra-articular corticosteroids are more given in the knee joint?
- Mode of injection
- Infrapatellar approach
- Suprapatellar approach
- Posterior approach
- Method of injecting into the anserinus bursa
- Osgood–Schlatter's disease (apophysitis of tibial tuberosity)
- How to aspirate knee joint?

Perhaps no other joint has been more popular a place for intra-articular injection than the knee joint, causes being:

1. The joint line is most easily felt and approachable and the joint spaces can be easily delineated percutaneously.
2. The knee joint is the most common site for degenerative changes, especially in the subjects with Asian culture. In these countries, social and religious obligations demand, quite often, squatting and sitting in **Budha's position** (crossed-legged position), which are definitely strenuous to the joints.
3. The articular surfaces being mostly flat, the injected drug rapidly spreads over, up to margins and easily baths the synovial surface.
4. Patients having affections of the knee, usually present quite early because being a direct weight bearing joint, even mild pain attracts the patient's attention instantaneously. In these stages of presentation, intra-articular injection of corticosteroid proves, in most of the circumstances, quite effective.

The most common indication of injecting corticoid or platelet-rich plasma is for osteoarthritis knee. However, in early cases the results after proximal fibular osteotomy appear better than even combined arthroscopically produced microfracture along with intraoperative autologous platelet-rich plasma.

MODE OF INJECTION

The joint can be approached anteriorly or posteriorly. However, anterior approaches being quite easy, are recommended. Anteriorly again, in the infra-patellar region medial or lateral joint spaces are easily negotiable. For the pathology localized mainly, in suprapatellar region; suprapatellar approaches, either from medial or lateral side (more easily approvable), can be more helpful.

INFRAPATELLAR APPROACH

Injection can be given either in sitting or lying down position. Since, in few cases, patients are sensitive to local anesthetics and a few patients are hypersensitive to any prick, it is better to give injections in lying down position.

Lying-down Position (Figure 12.1)

The patient lies supine. The knee is flexed to 60–80°. The tip of the index finger can be easily placed over anterior part of upper portion of tibial plateau over which the point of entry should be marked either by skin pencil or nail tip. Thence, after antiseptic preparations, the needle should be pushed backwards, with lateral or medial inclination correspondingly from inferomedial or inferolateral compartment, little above and parallel to the tibial plateau, till it is in the joint (which is indicated by loss of any resistance). It must be avoided to push too much within, as it may hurt the articular cartilage of femur, whereby the patient feels pain which may persist for a few days with or without swelling.

SUPRAPATELLAR APPROACH (FIGURE 12.2)

The patient lies supine. Knee is extended and the patient is asked to relax the quadriceps. The patella becomes lax and suprapatellar pouch also becomes loose. Palpate the superolateral or superomedial margin of the patella. Push the needle almost transversly a little above the upper margin of patella with slight upwards and posterior inclination. Try to avoid any contact with the bone. These approaches are usually recommended where there is some collection in suprapatellar pouch which makes the thrust of the needle markedly easier into the distended pouch. First, aspirate the collections. Corticosteroid should be only injected if the aspirate does not appear infected.

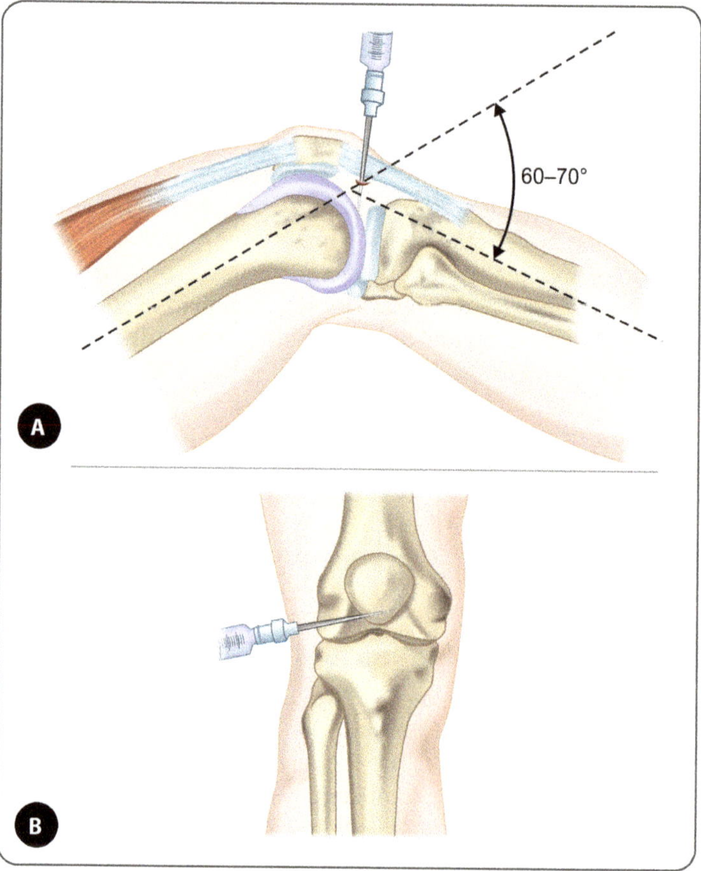

FIGS. 12.1A AND B: Knee joint—Infrapatellar approach in lying down position. Viewed from side (A); from above (B).

Sitting Position (Figure 12.3)

Only infrapatellar injections are recommended in this position. However, suprapatellar pricks can also be made, where there is collection in the suprapatellar pouch. In such cases, the knee is extended as far as practicable and the leg is supported over a sandbag placed behind the lower leg. For infrapatellar route, let the patient sit at the edge of the table with the leg hanging or resting on low stool; or on the chair with feet planted on the ground. The knee is flexed at about 90°. Locate the upper tibial plateau either laterally or medially and mark it with the nail-edge or skin pencil. After antiseptic cleaning push the needle directly posteriorly, little above and parallel to the tibial plateau with an inclination toward the mid-line.

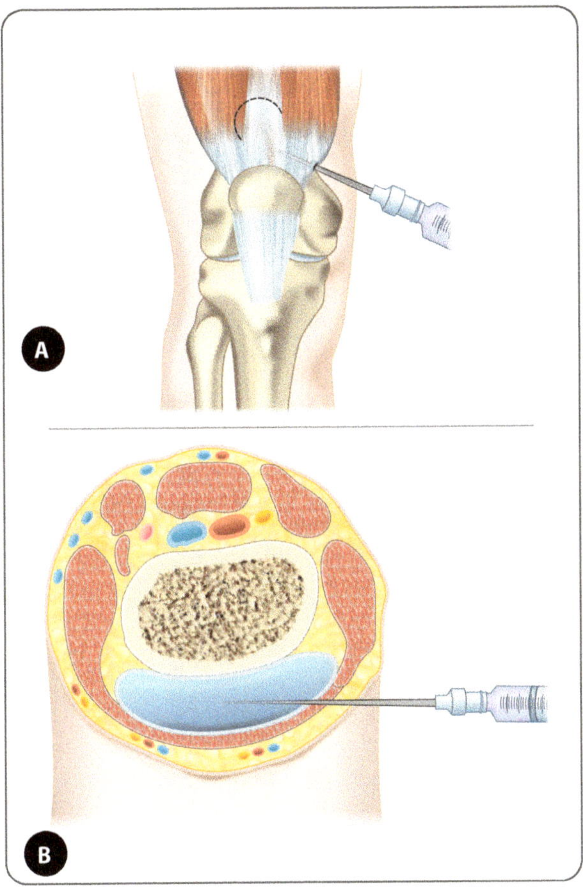

FIGS. 12.2A AND B: Knee joint—suprapatellar approach in lying down position. (A) Viewed from above; (B) Section showing needle into suprapatellar pouch.

POSTERIOR APPROACH

Posterior approaches are usually not recommended for intra-articular injections. In specific conditions, e.g., cysts from posterior part of semilunar cartilage, capsular cyst, **Morrant-Baker cyst** or any tender nonspecific condition in relation to posterior part of the knee, corticosteroid injection may be given by posterior approach. The cyst or spot to be pricked is approached directly, avoiding neurovascular bundle.

The bursae around the knee joint are also treated sometimes by injecting corticosteroid into them. These are more or less associated with the tendons around the knee joint. Any particular bursa can be palpated in relation to its tendon. It should be clearly delineated first and then pricked by direct approach. It is better to keep the needle inclined parallel to the corresponding tendon.

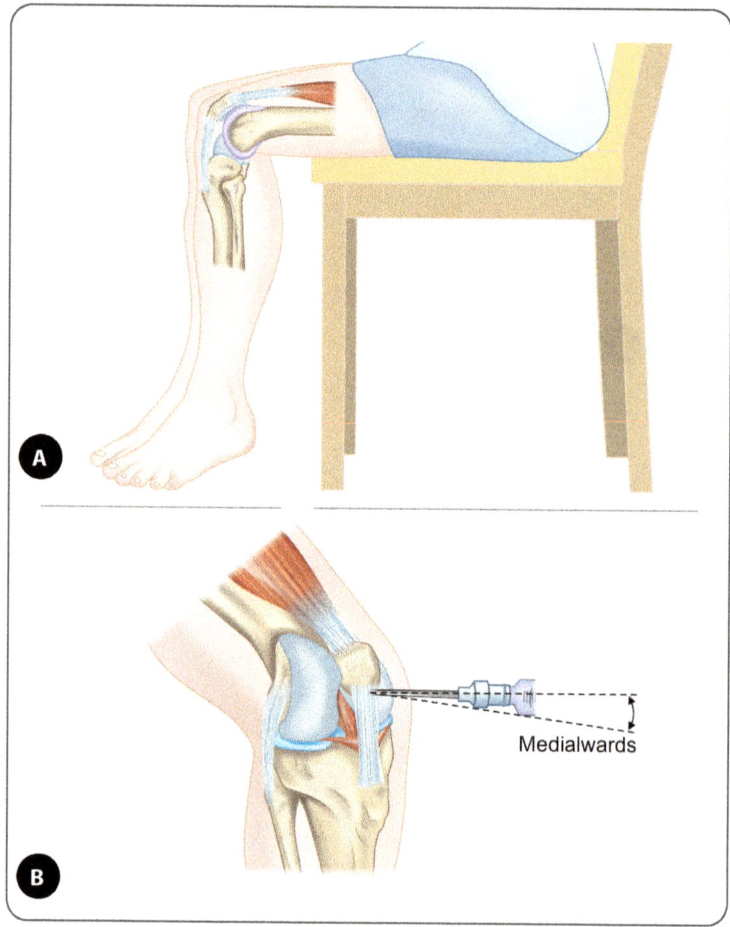

FIGS. 12.3A AND B: Knee joint—infrapatellar approach in sitting position.

In the management of the chronic bursitis of the anserinus bursa, infiltration of the corticosteroid is usually helpful.

METHOD OF INJECTING INTO THE ANSERINUS BURSA

The patient sits at the edge of the table. Palpate the medial side of the tibial crest below the patella. Note the tendinous attachment of the three muscles—(sartorius, gracilis and semitendinosus)—the pes anserinus. The anserinus bursa lies between the pes anserinus and the attachment of the medial collateral ligament of knee at the tibia. The injecting needle is directed parallel to pes anserinus attachment to reach the maximal tender point and swelling.

No Touch Technique of Injecting into the Knee Joint

To further improve the **NO TOUCH TECHNIQUE of intra-articular injection**, the point of injection can be selected visually as follows.

Place the tip of your left index finger on the top of the lateral tibial plateaux. About 0.75 cm above the corresponding point on the medial side of patellar ligament will be the point of inserting the needle on the infero-medial joint space. Similarly place the tip of left index finger on the top of medial tibial plateaux and the corresponding point on the parallel level on the lateral side of patellar ligament, will be the point of inserting the needle into the infralateral joint space. Similarly by fixing the patella with index finger the point of injecting on superomedial and superolateral region of patella can be visually fixed.

Injection Around/Into Lateral Popliteal Nerve

Corticosteroid is also used for infiltrating around and/or into the lateral popliteal nerve either for traumatic neuritis or Hansen's neuritis or for entrapment neuropathy **(Figure 12.4A)**.

The patient lies on the side, with the affected side above and the knee flexed by about 30°. Palpate lateral popliteal nerve below and behind the head of the fibula where it can be rolled against the neck of the fibula. Fixing the nerve at one point with the index finger, the perineural area is infiltrated with cocktail using a thin (22 bore) needle. The nerve can also be gently injected into, if required.

OSGOOD–SCHLATTER'S DISEASE (APOPHYSITIS OF TIBIAL TUBEROSITY)

Injection can be given either in lying down position or sitting position. Corticosteroid cocktail is infiltrated from either side just above the palpable upper limit of tibial tuberosity and just behind the ligamentum patellae. The needle is directed toward mid-line with slight posterior and downward inclination reaching just up to bony resistance **(Figure 12.4B)**.

HOW TO ASPIRATE KNEE JOINT?

The patient lies supine with knee slightly flexed (with leg placed on a rolled towel or a sandbag or a small pillow under the popliteal fossa, the patient can comfortably maintain workable degrees of flexion). After thoroughly cleaning and antiseptic preparation, the point of aspiration is visually fixed (not by touching) and infiltrated with the local anesthesia up to the joint capsule using a long 21–22 gauge needle. Then a 18 or 16 gauge aspiration needle is inserted just superior to the upper pole and just lateral to the lateral border of the patella at the level of the patellofemoral joint. The aspiration needle is directed horizontally and at right angles to the long axis of the limb. The needle should enter the joint capsule deep to the quadriceps tendon.

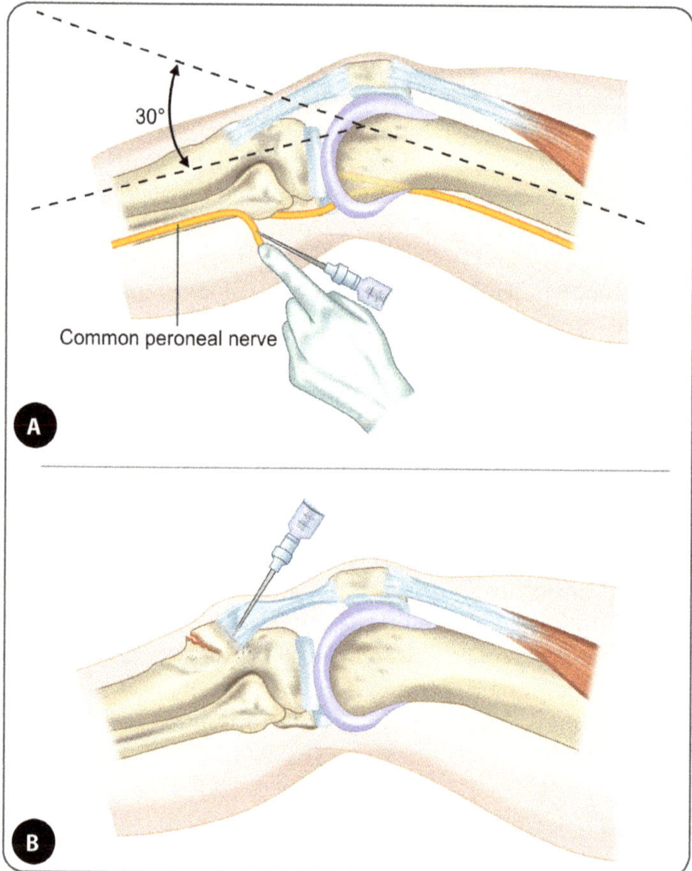

FIGS. 12.4A AND B: (A) Approach to lateral popliteal nerve; (B) Approach for Osgood-Schlatter's disease.

Fluid in the joint (most of the fluid remains in the suprapatellar pouch, which is always in continuation of the joint cavity) can be easily aspirated by 20–50 mL syringe. However, if there is difficulty in getting the fluid back—perhaps the needle is blocked by a bit of synovium or a flake of some diseased tissue—in such case, release the suction, move the bevel down or slightly in or out and try again. If the fluid initially comes out and then stops, ask the patient to contract quadriceps and slightly flex and extend the knee (most of the patients can do) or ask one assistant to press down on suprapatellar pouch by his/her hand using sterile gloves, thereby pushing the fluid into the joint cavity proper and then aspirate. After completing the aspiration take out the needle, put a sterile swab over the puncture-wound, do little massage with finger tip over the punctured zone to block the passage and seal the punctering passage from within and then seal the punctured point with tincture of benzoine or povidine iodine.

CHAPTER 13

Ankle Joint and Foot

"It takes half of your life before you discover life is a do-it-yourself project."

—**SP**

CHAPTER OUTLINE

- Indications
- Approaches
- Method of injection for different indications
- Painful heel syndrome
- Plantar fasciitis
- Symptomatic accessory navicular
- Subtalar joint

Ankle, on the whole, holds fewer indications for corticosteroid injection.

INDICATIONS

- Traumatic synovitis or arthritis
- Rheumatoid arthritis
- Degenerative arthritis
- **Crystal arthritis**
- **Gouty arthritis**
- **Ganglion in relation to ankle**

APPROACHES

Approaches are usually anterior. In other sides, the malleoli (medial, lateral and posterior) do overhang the joint to varying extents, and hence, it is very difficult to negotiate into the joint unless the joint capsule is distended.

METHOD OF INJECTION FOR DIFFERENT INDICATIONS

1. The patient lies supine. Place a sandbag behind the lower leg. In about 20–30° plantar flexed position of the ankle, the anterior joint margin

is widened and felt to some extent. Feel the pulsation of anterior tibial artery. Mark a point about a finger breadth on medial side or two fingers breadth on lateral side at which the needle is pushed posteriorly with 20° upward inclination. The needle enters without any resistance. Do avoid pricking through a tendon **(Figure 13.1)**.

2. The patient lies in the same position as in the above method. Put the index finger just anterior to medial malleolus. With passive movements of the ankle, joint margin can be felt to varying extent, keep that position of the ankle in which the joint space is felt maximum. Push the needle posteriorly with upwards and lateral inclination. Avoid hitting the articular cartilage.

In the ankle region, tenosynovitis of tibialis posterior and peroneal tendons require corticosteroid injection. However, any tendon in that region can have this pathology.

Tibialis Posterior

It sometimes suffers from nonspecific inflammatory changes which often cause pain in that region, that also gets relieved to a varying extent with corticosteroid injection.

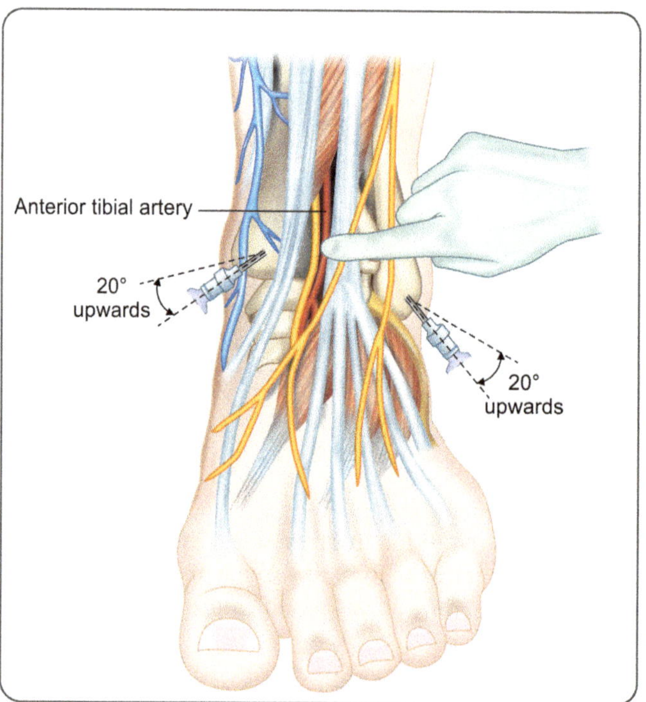

FIG. 13.1: Ankle joint—anterior approach.

Method (Figure 13.2)

The tibialis posterior tendon stands prominent when patient actively plantar-flexes and inverts the foot simultaneously. The tendon is located from above and then while coursing behind the medial malleolus. Keeping the needle almost parallel to the tendon in that site, it can be pushed upward with a slight lateral and posterior inclination.

The patient lies supine with dorsolateral aspect of the forefoot supported over a sandbag. The ankle automatically goes in the attitude of plantar flexion and inversion. The needle enters into the sheath, which should be confirmed as follows:

- Keep the needle engaged into the supposed sheath. Detach the syringe and ask the patient to relax and then invert the foot repeatedly. With every action of the inversion, the needle moves up and down with tibialis posterior tendon.

Peroneus Longus

Besides tenosynovitis, peroneal spasm leading to spasmodic flat foot also responds to corticosteroid injection many a times.

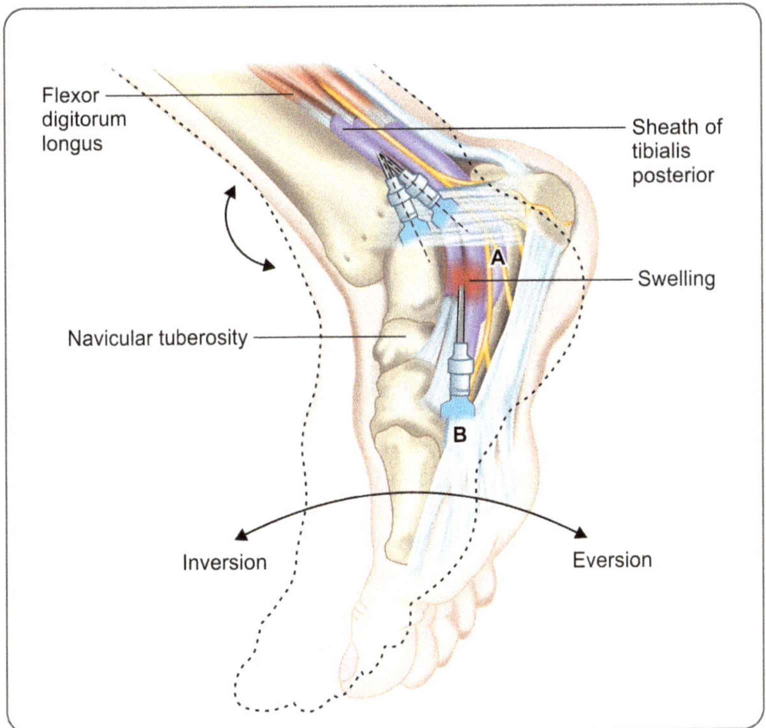

FIG. 13.2: (A) Approach to tibialis posterior tendon; (B) Approach for accessory navicular.

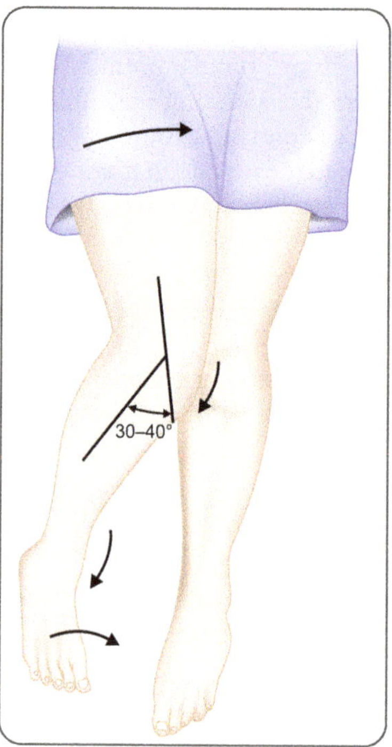

FIG. 13.3: Position of patient for injecting into tendon sheath of peroneus longus.

Method (Figures 13.3 and 13.4)

The patient lies supine, keeping his affected lower limb 30° flexed and fully internally rotated at hip. The knee is flexed by 30–40°. This position can be easily held by putting a sandbag beneath the buttock of the affected side. Keep another sandbag beneath the lower leg. Locate the tendon posterosuperior to lateral malleolus by asking the patient to plantar-flex and evert the foot simultaneously. Keeping the needle almost parallel to the tendon at the located site, it is pushed posteriorly with upwards and medial inclination. It enters into the sheath. Test by detaching the syringe and asking the patient to actively plantar-flex and evert the foot. With the action of tendon, the needle moves up and down.

Sometimes, ganglions in relation to ankle joint or surrounding tendons are treated by directly injecting corticosteroid or cocktail.

PAINFUL HEEL SYNDROME (FIGURE 13.5)

In painful heel, the complain of pain and tenderness hovers around the anteromedial prominence of the calcaneal tuberosity. The exact cause of this clinical entity is hardly known. Probably inferring on it Stiell (1922) stated, *"Painful heel appears to be a condition which is seldom efficiently*

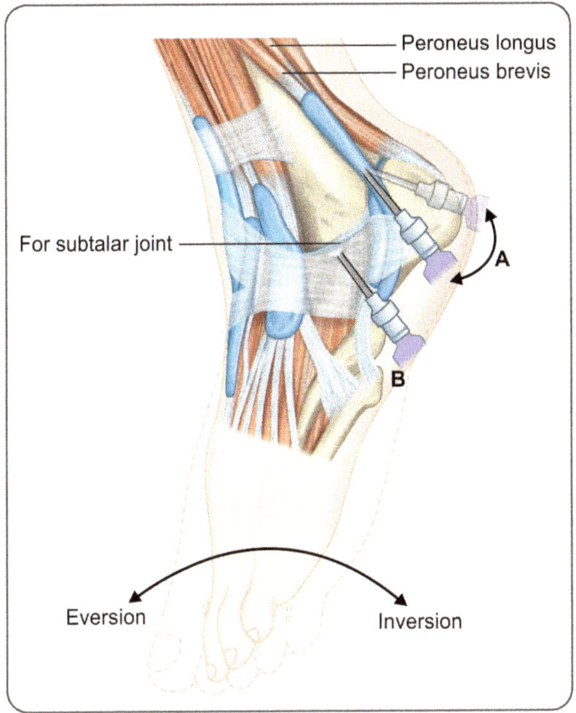

FIG. 13.4: (A) Approach to peroneus longus tendon; (B) Approach for subtalar joint.

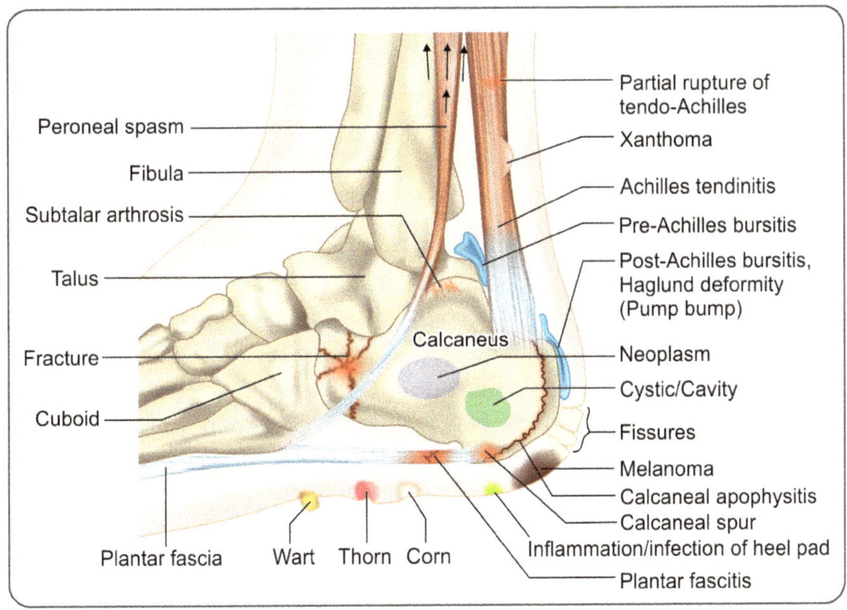

FIG. 13.5: Usual causes of pain in and around the heel (Painful heel syndrome).

treated, for the simple reason that the causation is not exactly diagnosed." The broad mechanisms to explain the causes of nonspecific painful heel have been considered as: (i) Degenerative process in the calcaneal heel pad; (ii) **Windless mechanism of the plantar fascia** with the dorsiflexion of the toes; the most dense tight portion of planter fascia/aponeurosis originates from the anteromedial aspect of calcaneal tuberosity which is also the most common tender site located during clinical examination; (iii) The entrapment of the first branch of lateral planter nerve to abductor digiti minimi (between the deep surface of the flexor digitorum brevis and the heel spur and adjacent quadratus plantae muscle) has been found as a possible neurogenic cause of painful heel syndrome.

Pain in the heel region has been a common complain due to various reasons.

The common conditions requiring corticosteroid injections are:

1. **Pre-Achilles bursitis**
2. **Haglund deformity (Pump bump)**—it is caused by chronic inflammation of the **adventitious superficial pretendinous Achilles bursa**
3. **Post-Achilles bursitis**
4. **Achilles tendinitis**
5. **Calcaneal apophysitis**
6. **Plantar fasciitis—the most common cause of heel pain**
7. **Calcaneal spur syndrome, etc.**

Nonspecific inflammatory conditions around the tendo-Achilles are usually the cause of pain in the back of heel. They may be associated with a swelling of varying consistency in relation to the lowest part of Achilles tendon. Most of the patients present for treatment only when they are symptomatic.

Injection can be given from any side of the tendo-Achilles. The patient lies on the side with mid-leg supported on a sandbag, so that Achilles tendon region remains free from any contact for cleaning from all around. The needle is pushed at a point of maximum tenderness either anteriorly or posteriorly to the tendo-Achilles depending upon whether it is for pre-Achilles or post-Achilles condition **(Figure 13.6)**.

In the calcaneal apophysitis (in early adolescent age group), the symptoms are quite often relieved by infiltration of corticosteroid. The injection should be given into the lowest insertion of tendo-Achilles from either side, better from outer one. The position and method are same as for Achilles-bursitis. However, boots with raised and softly padded heel top platform should also be recommended alongwith, in such pathologies in and around the Achilles tendon.

PLANTAR FASCIITIS

Plantar fasciitis is localized inflammation and degeneration of plantar aponeurosis. It is the most common cause of plantar heel pain. The patient

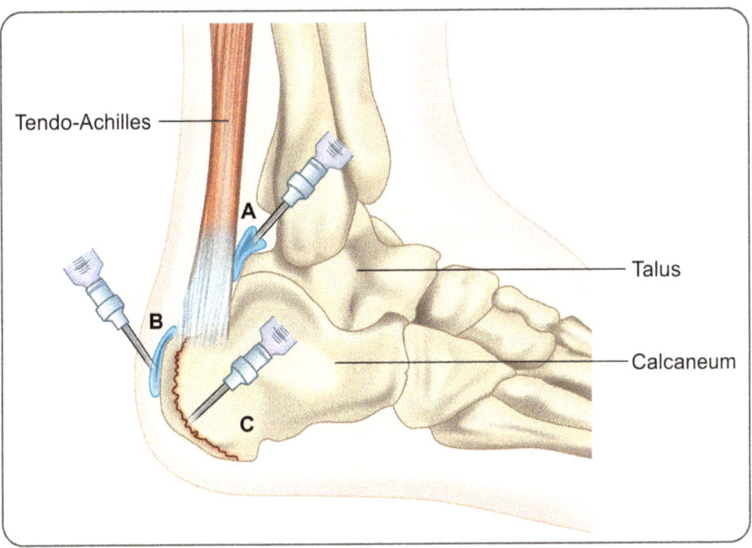

FIG. 13.6: Site of injection for (A) Pre-Achilles bursitis; (B) Post-Achilles bursitis; (C) Calcaneal apophysitis.

lies supine, with lower leg supported over a sandbag. The leg is kept in externally rotated position **(Figure 13.7A)**. In plantar fasciitis, usually the most painful spot is located by pressing with the fingertip toward the under surface of calcaneum on the inferomedial aspect of the sole part of heel at the region from where medial arch takes an upward curve. With a fingertip, this area should be localized by direct pressure. The needle is pushed into the region of maximum tenderness with an inclination backwards, outwards and slightly upwards for about 2.5 cm. Posterior attachment of plantar fascia is usually engaged into, which requires infiltration. By pushing the needle a little outwards the drug can be injected for calcaneal spur syndrome **(Figure 13.7B)**. Accurate targeting of the spot—calcaneal spur point (proximal attachment of the plantar fascia to the medical tubercle of the tuberosity of calcaneum) for corticosteroid injection is essential to achieve proper effect. Platelet-rich plasma (PRP) injection appears to be more effective than corticosteroid for reduction of pain. However, both PRP and corticoids are safe and effective treatment options for chronic plantar fasciitis. Salvi (2015) has suggested to use lateral radiograph of foot to target the plantar fascia. On lateral X-ray the spur is targeted by two intersecting lines—one drawn tangent to the posterior margin of medial malleolus and parallel to the long axis of tibia with the foot near a right angle to the leg. The second line is drawn tangent to the plantar surface of the tuberosity of calcaneum and parallel to the substrate. The corresponding lines can be drawn on the skin surface to locate the intersection point at which the needle should be inserted. In most of the patients symptoms resolve with conservative treatment. However, in a small group of patients, mechanical

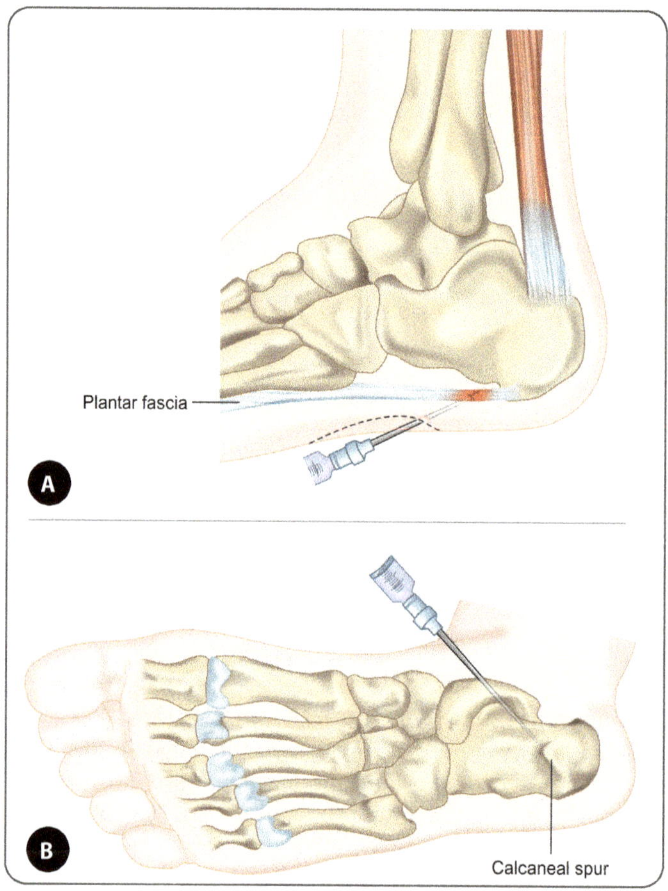

FIGS 13.7A AND B: (A) Section showing approach for plantar fasciitis; (B) Approach for calcaneal spur.

perturbations (equinus, aponeurotic thickening, loss of tissue elasticity) and increased hydrostatic tissue pressures, reduce vascular flows and initiate a noninflammatory degenerative process referred to as refractory plantar fasciitis (RPF) (Rushing G et al. 2020) RPF patients were treated with bipolar radiofrequency-controlled ablation with/and PRP injection. Majority of these patients had highly satisfactory results and their long-term outcomes remained comparable to that after plantar fasciotomy.

Electromagnetically generated extracorporeal shock wave therapy (ESWT) is being successfully used for plantar fasciitis as well like other orthopedic indications, e.g., calcified tendonitis of the shoulder, Achilles and patellar tendinopathies, lateral epicondylitis, etc. This therapy utilizes shock waves (about 240 per minute)—using electromagnetic shock wave emitter (EMSE) power source versus power source technology—utilizes shock waves which can penetrate even up to 7.5 cm to trigger the body's own repair mechanisms and overstimulate pain transmission nerves. This therapy is safe, effective and efficient, and a high number of shock waves (about 240 per minutes) reduce sensitivity and pain.

Computer-controlled local anesthetic (or other agents) delivery system (CompuMed) is a revolutionary system which allows to easily deliver virtually painfree injection in conditions such as heel spur syndrome, plantar fasciitis, neuroma, metatarsalgia, hallux blocks, etc.

Other conditions of foot requiring corticosteroid injections are:

- Symptomatic accessory navicular, bunion in relation to the head of first metatarsal, metatarsalgia, entrapment of 2nd or 3rd interdigital nerves, painful warts, collagen arthropathy, gouty arthritis, especially of metatarsophalangeal and interphalangeal joints (in rheumatoid arthritis and gouty arthritis) tendovaginitis of tibialis posterior and into peroneal sheath.

SYMPTOMATIC ACCESSORY NAVICULAR (SEE FIGURE 13.2)

Patient's position will be the same as for injecting into tibialis posterior sheath. Feel navicular tuberosity. Accessory navicular usually lies posteroinferior to it. Infiltrate around this knob-like swelling by direct approach. For osteochondritis of navicular (Kohler's disease) and any other tarsal bone, similar infiltrations around the affected zone work quite satisfactorily and give symptomatic relief.

SUBTALAR JOINT

Following fracture calcaneum, which usually involves subtalar joint in most of the cases, traumatic subtalar arthrosis is a common complication. The patient keeps on feeling pain in subtalar region for 4–5 years, or even more. Usually, walking on the uneven ground or sudden inversion or eversion of foot or keeping foot suddenly on the edge of the step initiates or aggravates the pain. Quite often this condition responds symptomatically to corticosteroid infiltration.

Method (see Figure 13.4)

Injection can be given with the patient either lying down supine or sitting with foot hanging. It is better with the patient lying down. Patient lies supine with hip flexed 30° and fully internally rotated. The knee is flexed 30–40°. The lower leg is supported on a sandbag. The foot has tendency to go for inversion and plantar flexion. Antero-infero-medial to lateral malleolus, the gap of sinus tarsi can be felt. Push the needle directly into the gap medially with slight posterior and upward inclination. The needle enters the region of subtalar joint without any resistance. Also, infiltrate into the sinus tarsi simultaneously.

CHAPTER 14

Spine, Peripheral Nerves, Sacroiliac Joint

"Corruption is like a ball of snow, once it's set A-rolling it must increase."

—Charles Caleb Cotton

CHAPTER OUTLINE

- Injections for low back pain
- Herpetic neuritis
- Lumbar disc disease
- Epidural steroid injections
- Complications of epidural injections
- Selective nerve root injection
- Method of nerve root injection
- Vertebroplasty and kyphoplasty
- Injection into and around the peripheral nerves
- How to inject into and around the ulnar nerve?
- How to inject into and around the lateral popliteal nerve?
- How to inject around the lateral cutaneous nerve of thigh?
- Coccydodynia (painful coccyx)
- Infiltration into and around sciatic nerve
- Old pelvic fracture
- Recurrent fibrositis
- Rheumatoid spondylitis
- Sacroiliac joint

In chronic back and neck pain, not amenable to various noninvasive mode of management like NSAIDs, postural adjustments, physiotherapy, manipulations, traction, heat therapy, TENS, inferential therapy, etc., injections of corticosteroids (locally into the facet joint, in and around the root, trigger points, etc.) may prove useful. In radicular pain locate the desired root, reproduce the pain, block the pain and inject steroid. Generation of trigger spot is mediated through neurogenic impulse and it can behave as an ectopic pain source. Hence, to achieve good result, it is worthwhile to block trigger spots along with the respective root/facet/epidural block. The injection can be given with more precision under the image intensifier. The suspected pain sources should be injected one by one with post-injection clinical assessment done after each injection. Different concentrations of anesthetic agents (e.g., Xylocaine) are used to block different types of neural fibres, such as: 0.5% for sympathetic fibres; 1% for sensory fibres; 2% for motor fibres.

INJECTIONS FOR LOW BACK PAIN

In managing low back pain, injection treatment is used in three forms according to the indications:

1. Trigger point injection
2. Facet joint injection
3. Epidural corticosteroid injection

Myofascial trigger points, though remain controversial, are frequently diagnosed and injection of anesthetic agents and corticosteroids into and around these points do help in several cases. However, it is not clear to what extent the efficacy of trigger point injection exceeds that of placebo effects.

Facet joints pathologies, especially degenerative ones, have been a source of chronic low back pain. The facet joint syndrome is more common in elderly people. Clinically, there is no pathognomonic diagnostic feature of this syndrome. It can be only confirmed by obtaining relief of pain after fluoroscopic-guided local anesthetic block of joint or its nerve supply. Once origin of pain is localized in the facet joint it can be treated either by intra-articular injection of corticosteroid or percutaneous ablation of the nerve supply to the joint. The response, to either of two, is up to moderate extent.

If taken together right from cervical to lumbosacral, the degenerative changes involve the spinal column most frequently. For similar conditions in the limb joints, corticosteroid injection has been considered as an effective drug for providing symptomatic relief. But, for the spinal joints, this mode of management could not get firm ground; probably, due to the fact that the joints are comparatively deeply placed and their approaches are circuitous. For conditions like strain, sprain and fibrosistis involving the supra- and interspinous ligaments, the corticosteroids' cocktail injections have been frequently effective. The best guide is to inject at the site of maximum tenderness and the adjoining areas.

Epidural injections in the cervical, thoracic and lumbosacral spine have been given to diagnose, localize and treat spinal pain.

HERPETIC NEURITIS

Corticosteroid may be effective if injected properly around the involved root. However, this is not a very easy procedure. The patient lies on lateral side, with the side to be injected below. One has to use a comparatively long slender needle, and to select the particular root course. Along this course, at about 3.5 cm outside the midspinal line, start with the inclination of the needle up medially and anteriorly along the lower costal margin. Local anesthetic should be infiltrated first along the course of needle. The moment, proper root is cuffed around by the local anesthetic agent, the patient's burning sensation and pain will be lessened to a varying extent. Then, the corticosteroid cocktail is injected at that site and also for some distance while withdrawing the needle **(Figure 14.1A)**.

LUMBAR DISC DISEASE (FIGURE 14.1B)

In lumbar disc, the role of corticosteroid is variable. It is also not that easy to inject into the disc. This should better be done under the image intensifier. However, in the inflamed state of the disc, help rendered by the corticosteroid cocktail, either by virtue of producing a dent into the tense discoid space or by anti-inflammatory action is debatable. Further, the inflamed root, if injected appropriately, have been seen to respond well. For prolapsed intervertebral disc, the role of chymopapain has been seen to be more effective, if injected into the disc in earlier stage. **Chymopapain**, a proteolytic enzyme, can dissolve specifically the nucleus in the intervertebral disc. The process is known as chemonucleolysis. However, this injection must be given by an experienced hand intradiscally under the image intensifier.

For **discography** some safe contrast media, such as **diatrizoate meglumine (Hypaque), iothalamate meglumine (conray), iohexol (omnipaque), metrizamide (Amipaque)** and **iopamidol** may be used, however, one should be cautious and ready for any possible complication.

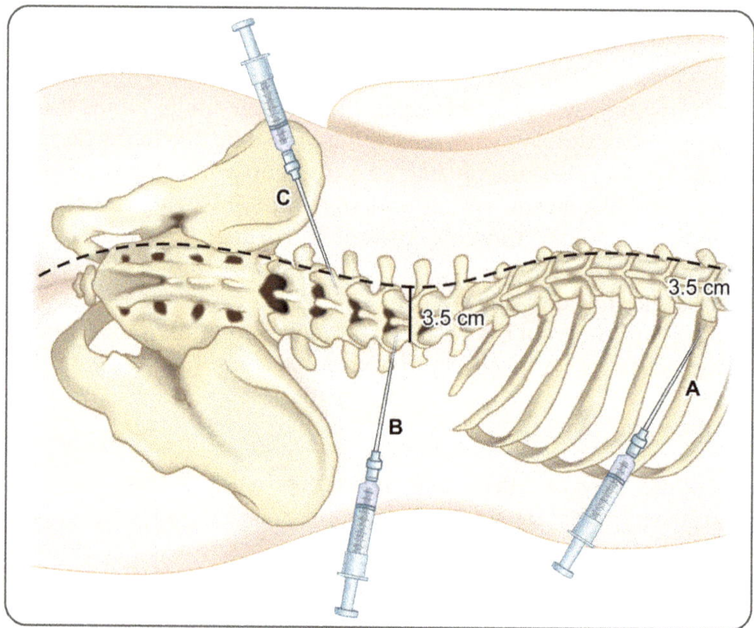

FIGS. 14.1A TO C: Sites of injection. (A) For herpetic neuritis in thoracic region; (B) For lumbar-disc disease; (C) Intrathecally through lumbar puncture (LP) route.

Anatomy

The epidural space (extradural space, peridural space) is the space between the two layers of the dura mater formed by its division at the edge of the foramen magnum. The outer layer forms like periosteum of the vertebral column and the inner, the actual spinal dura mater. The epidural space is limited caudally by the sacrococcygeal ligament. It contains a number of venous plexus as well as fat and connective tissue.

EPIDURAL STEROID INJECTIONS

Epidural injections were developed to diagnose and treat pain in the cervical, thoracic, lumbar and lumbosacral regions. These injections are invariably used to relive pain in acute disc pathology and nerve root injuries. The transforaminal epidural injection appears to have better short term pain relief in discogenic radiculopathy. However, in cervical and lumbar regions interlaminar and caudal epidural injections have been found to be effective in relieving chronic discogenic pain with or without radiculitis.

Epidural steroid injections were used to treat local back-pain with associated sciatica due to disc herniation since 1950s. In disc prolapse, the inflammatory reactions develop invariably. In such inflammation locally applied corticosteroids have their effect on membrane stabilization and antinociceptive C-fibres and their interference with neuropeptide and inflammatory mediator activities (Johansson et al. 1990). Now it has become an integral part of nonsurgical management of low back pain providing relief from 1 week to 1 year or even more. On overall assessment about 50% of patients get relief. The short-term benefits have been uniformly seen, however, these injections, usually, do not alter long-term outcomes. Caudal epidural can be given through sacral hiatus, interlaminar or transforaminal route.

For epidural injections the steroids preparation containing betamethasone sodium phosphate and betamethasone acetate (such as celestone soluspan) has been found to act fast with long-lasting result. It should be given alone. It should not be mixed with any local anesthetic containing preservatives like parabens or phenol to avoid any flocculation and clogging of the suspension. Other steroids used for epidural injection are methylprednisolone (Depo-Medrol) and triamcinolone acetonide (Kenalog). Steroids may be used with isotonic saline or the later may be used alone in good volume (60–80 mL) epidurally (at least through sacral hiatus route). This volume of isotonic saline baths around the affected spinal roots and separate them from any adhesion in the intervertebral root canal.

Singla et al. (2017) in a study over the patients of symptomatic lumbar stenosis undergoing lumbar epidural steroid injection prior to surgical decompression have observed that there may be at an increased risk of post operative wound infection.

Principle

The drug, to be effective, must be infiltrated around the affected nerve root.

Indications

- Cases of resistant radiculitis which have not responded to adequate conservative treatment
- The cases, which have frequent recurrences
- Annoying persistence of radicular symptoms for pretty long time with fluctuations
- Epidural methylprednisolone enhances overall recovery after discectomy for herniated disc including reduction of neurological impairment.

Indications for epidural steroid injection **in cervical region** are discogenic radiculopathies, cervical spondylosis of disc degeneration origin, cervicobrachial neurologics, myofacial pain, cervical strains, reflex sympathetic dystrophy, post-herpatic neuralgia, etc. There may be inadvertent injection into radicular artery or even vertebral artery, hence cervical route should be avoided. **In the thoracic region** epidural steroid injection is given for discogenic radicular pain, traumatic neuropathy, herpes zoster, idiopathic thoracic neuralgia, etc. **In lumbar region** main indications are discogenic radicular pain, lateral root canal stenosis, or nerve injury radicular pain.

In any region, depending upon the expertise of surgeon and available facilities, the route of injection can be chosen—interlaminar, or transforaminal. For **lower lumbar region** sacral hiatus route is also available.

Mode of Injections

Diagnostic or therapeutic epidural injections should be preferably given under fluoroscopic control since:

1. Accuracy of injection site is more achieved, i.e., the needle goes accurately in epidural space or the intended interspace. Even in experienced hands the misplacement of needle is about 30%, if given without fluoroscopic control.
2. The possibility of accidental intravascular injection is avoided. Without fluoroscopy, the anatomical anomalies like midline epidural septum or multiple separate epidural compartments cannot be detected, which if present restricts the flow of injected material to the desired place.

Through Sacral Hiatus (Figure 14.2)

The patient lies prone with legs kept extended and with a pillow or sandbag beneath the pubic symphisis. Feel the fused spinous process of sacrum. Slip the index finger gradually down the fused spinous processes. Suddenly, inverted U-shaped deficiency of the sacral hiatus with curved sharp margin on the sides—sacral cornua can be felt. Infiltrate local anesthetic

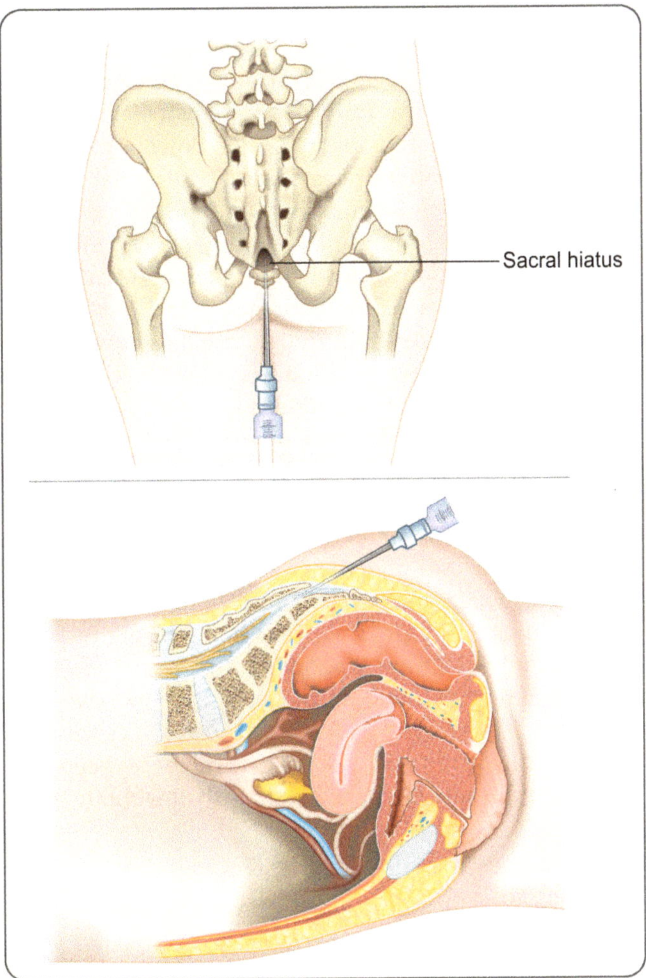

FIG. 14.2: Epidural injection through sacral hiatus. Above—viewed from above, Below—sagittal section showing needle in position.

at the hiatus. After waiting for two minutes (to observe for any reaction and for anesthetic action effect), a sterile no: 20 lumbar puncture needle is introduced through the hiatus, with beveled edge grazing over the bone, after holding the skin tight by the thumb and index finger or index and middle fingers of the opposite hand. Straight needle is usually used, but it is preferable to use bent needle, which facilitates the negotiating of the needle. After negotiating the sacral canal for about 2.5–3.5 cm, a feeling of slight yielding can be felt, then stop pushing the needle. Pull the piston of the syringe. If the needle has entered into the epidural space, an effortless pulling will be observed and a negative pressure is created in the syringe; and after leaving the piston it returns to the end. The stellate is removed and leakage of any cerebrospinal fluid is watched. After confirming that no cerebrospinal fluid was coming out, and there is no resistance in pushing 3-5 cc of air within, inject 50 mL of normal saline with 30-160 mg of methylprednisolone very slowly. Initially, the patient may feel some pain but very soon it settles down. Let the patient settle down. Again after injecting about 30-40 mL of fluid patient feels some bursting pain due to volume injected. Keeping the needle-syringe in situ, pause for a while, the pain settles down. Then complete the injection very slowly. After withdrawing the needle, the injecting point is slowly massaged and sealed with tincture of benzoin or povidonc iodine. The patient is asked to turn on side, with the lower limb, to which pain was radiating, lying down. The patient is transferred to bed in lying down position with raised head. The head end of the bed is raised so that the injected fluid remains confined to the affected zone as long as possible and the patient is advised to rest for 12 hours. Usually, the patient starts feeling better by 2-4 hours. Usually, one prick is considerably effective, however, depending upon the symptoms, injection may be repeated fortnightly or at monthly intervals. If one injection is totally ineffective, no further injection should be given. It is reasonable to perform up to 3-4 injections per year. The patient should take rest on the day of injection. Epidural steroid injection should be combined with usual physiotherapy and rehabilitation programs.

The transforaminal epidural injection appears to have better short-term pain relief in discogenic radiculopathy. However, cervical and lumbar interlaminar and caudal epidural injection—all have been found to be effective in relieving chronic discogenic pain with or without radiculitis.

Through Lumbar Puncture Route (Figure 14.1C)

The patient should lie with the affected side of the root being low. Select the particular space according to the route involvement. Do the lumbar puncture with cautious push so that the subarachnoid space is not entered into, i.e., stops just short of it. After the lumbar puncture needle enters the dura, take out the stylet, connect the syringe. The piston can be pulled effortlessly when the desired subdural space is reached. Inject the local anesthetic after the appropriate position is reached. Ensure that the head end (with chest raised) to avoid the travelling of anesthetic agent upward from the desired place. If the right position is selected, pain is markedly reduced. Inject 40-80 mg of methylprednisolone along with 40-50 mL of normal saline. The patient lies for some time (half an hour) in this position.

Injection from the Lumbar Route

Injection can also be given through the lumbar root. The patient lies on the side to be injected below. The course of a particular root is assessed 3.5 cm outside the midspine line, the needle is pushed, with an inclination upwards, medially and slightly anteriorly to aim at the intervertebral foramina. Negotiating the needle along the intervertebral foramina corticosteroid should be injected. Working under image intensifier will markedly facilitate the injection.

Injection into Facet Joints (Zygapophyseal Joint)

Problems of facet joints have been a source of variable degrees of pain in the back. The involvement of facet may be due to various causes like synovial and/or capsular involvements, chondromalacic changes in facets, synovial impingement, injury to capsule, osteoarthritis, etc. Except for suspicion from clinical history and examination, it is difficult to pin-point the pathology in the facet joint as a cause of back pain. Once the cause of back pain is pin-pointed in the facet joint, noninvasive conservative management must be exhausted before going for fluoroscopically guided injection of corticosteroid into the facet joint. In cervical region, facet joint injection should be given in prone position under fluoroscopy.

COMPLICATIONS OF EPIDURAL INJECTIONS

Complications of these injections may be headache, dizziness, transient local pain, tingling, numbness, nausea and rarely infection.

As acute complication there may be vasovagal attack. With cautious approach the dural puncture is rare, and that too in cervical or lumbar route injections. Post injection headache may occur even if dura has not been punctured. However, headache may occur due to overenthusiastic or inadvertent injection of air, unrecognized mild dural puncture, increased intrathecal pressure due to injected fluid around the dural sac.

Locally dural puncture infection and arachnoiditis can occur. Preservative free solutions and fluoroscopy should be used to minimize arachnoiditis. Systemically, there are certain potential risks of treatment such as decrease in immunity, hyperglycemia, gastric ulcers, avascular necrosis, etc.

Epidural injections act by inducing steroids directly to the painful root to help in decreasing the inflammation. There may also be flushing effect by removing or flushing out inflammatory proteins causing pain.

Notable serious complications, though very few, like epidural hematoma, epidural abscess, durocutaneous fistula, Cushing syndrome may occur. Most of the possible acute or chronic complications can be avoided with proper antiseptic care and by injecting in fluoroscopy suit equipped with resuscitative and monitoring measure. Patient should be with intravenous cathetor intact before entering the operation theater.

Since I Macnab (1971) described the technique of nerve root injection for radioculopathy, it has been found to be effective for radicular pain. Epidural injection of steroids is a popular method for managing lumbar radioculopathy, but has not been commonly used for root injections at thoracic and thoraco-lumbar levels, due to possible neurological complications.

SELECTIVE NERVE ROOT INJECTION

The term coined by JF Krempen and BS Smith in 1974 has been used diagnostically or to predict the outcome of surgery. Therapeutic efficiency of nerve root injection has been well-proved in radicular pain caused by intervertebral disc herniation and discogenic spinal stenosis even to the extent of obviating the need for an operation in more than half of the patients in whom surgery would have been recommended. Nerve-root injections (mixture of 0.5 mL of 2% lidocaine, 0.5 mL of 0.5% bupivacaine and 40 mg of Depo-Medrol) are also effective in the treatment of pain resulting from osteoporotic vertebral fractures. It must be tried in patients with refractory pain from osteoporotic vertebral fractures before considering percutaneous vertebroplasty—percutaneous injection of poly(methylmethacrylate) (PMMA) into the vertebral bodies to augment the osteoporotic vertebral bodies, or any operative intervention (Don-Jun Kim et al. 2003).

METHOD OF NERVE ROOT INJECTION

It must be done under the image intensifier. The patient lies prone. After preparing the back skin, the site of the introduction of the needle is localized by the tip of a sterile artery forceps placed at the point of intersection between the lateral margin of the lamina and the inferior margin of the transverse process (as visualized in the fluoroscopy/image intensifier). This site of entry is marked with indelible ink. After infiltrating 1% lidocain, a 20-gauge, 13 cm spinal needle is inserted under fluoroscopic guidance into the selected intervertebral foramen. When the nerve root is touched, the patient feels a sharp radiating pain almost reproducing the symptom pain (which he/she was feeling earlier). After confirming by the reproduction of the symptom, the mixture of 0.5 mL of 2% lidocaine, 0.5 mL of 0.5% bupivacaine and 40 mg depomedrol is slowly injected.

The injection can be repeated at 2 weeks intervals to a maximum of three or until there was symptomatic improvement. While using nerve-root injection for fractures, too much of steroids must be avoided (maximum of 100 mg).

VERTEBROPLASTY AND KYPHOPLASTY

Vertebroplasty was first performed in 1984 for the treatment of cervical vertebral hemangioma in France. To augment the grossly osteoporosed (rarefied) painful collapsing vertebrae **PMMA** is injected percutaneously under the image intensifier into the osteoporotic vertebral bodies.

The technique is easy and fairly effective in most of the patients in providing relief from pain besides immediate good mechanical results. However, certain possible complications must always be kept in mind such as cell death caused by high polymerization temperature of PMMA; leakage of PMMA in the adjacent structures; differences in mechanical strength of the injected vertebrae compared with the adjacent ones, etc. Further, the long-term biocompatibility of PMMA is jeopardized by its presence as a permanent implant.

INJECTION INTO AND AROUND THE PERIPHERAL NERVES

Indications are few such as Hansen's neuritis, traumatic adhesion of nerve, early gliosis, entrapment neuropathy (of various nerves at various sites). Common nerves infiltrated are ulnar nerve in and above the medial epicondylar groove; lateral popliteal nerve at and proximal to the neck of fibula; lateral cutaneous nerve of thigh (meralgia paresthetica) just inferomedial to anterior superior iliac spine.

In entrapment neuropathy, the corticosteroid cocktail should be injected around the nerve in the compressive canal (fibro-osseous or intertendinous or inter-musculo-fibrous band).

In Hansen's neuropathy, the corticosteroid should be injected into and around the affected nerve. Ulnar and lateral popliteal nerves are mostly affected in Hansen's disease, followed by posterior auricular nerve, lateral cutaneous nerve of thigh, etc.

HOW TO INJECT INTO AND AROUND THE ULNAR NERVE?

The ulnar nerve is affected in the cubital tunnel and above it on the posteromedial aspect of lower and lower mid-arm—where the tender nerve thickening can be well-appreciated.

Method

The patient lies semisupine with affected side arm externally rotated and elbow flexed by 45°. One assistant holds that upper limb by one hand and keeps it steady by holding it at upper part of arm. After preparing from mid-arm to mid-forearm, the needle is introduced around the most palpable ulnar nerve and the prepared corticosteroid cocktail is infiltrated around the nerve. Then, in case of Hansen's neuritis, the needle is little withdrawn and then gently pushed into the substance of the nerve (easy resistance) and the cocktail is injected. After the needle is withdrawn, the patient is asked to flex and extend the elbow a few times.

HOW TO INJECT INTO AND AROUND THE LATERAL POPLITEAL NERVE?

The patient lies semisupinated with the affected side lower limb flexed at hip by 40° and internally rotated by 30° and flexed at knee by 45°. The lateral popliteal nerve can be palpated and rolled on the outer side of neck of fibula and above it. Injection is made around the nerve at and above the neck of the fibula and into the nerve just proximal to the neck of fibula. After withdrawing the needle, the patient is asked to flex and extend the knee a few times.

HOW TO INJECT AROUND THE LATERAL CUTANEOUS NERVE OF THIGH?

The patient lies supine with a thin sandbag placed beneath the hemipelvis on which side the lateral cutaneous nerve of thigh is to be injected. After antiseptic preparation, a point is located, one finger breadth below and medial to the anterior superior iliac spine, in which zone the lateral cutaneous nerve of thigh lies after emerging from beneath the outer end of inguinal ligament. The needle is pushed with upward inclination of about 30° at the selected point for about 1–1.5 cm depth. The prepared corticosteroid cocktail is infiltrated in that zone in about 1.5 cm radius. If the injection has been properly given, the patient will have anesthesia/ hypoesthesia in the palm size area on anterolateral aspect of thigh in middle and lower 1/3rd junctional zone. However, the patient might have disturbed sensation (hyperesthesia or hypoesthesia) in that zone from beforehand due to entrapment of the lateral cutaneous nerve of thigh.

COCCYDODYNIA (PAINFUL COCCYX)

For the coccygeal pain without any organic lesion (e.g., due to some pelvic pathology or neoplastic conditions) local infiltration of corticosteroid cocktail has been observed to be frequently effective.

Method (Figure 14.3A)

The patient lies either in fully prone position with a pillow beneath symphysis pubis or in lateral position. At the lowest end of the sacrum in the natal cleft, the needle is pushed anteriorly with downward inclination, grazing along one margin of the coccyx. The drug is pushed in tip region and around the coccyx as far as practicable. Similar process is repeated on the contralateral side keeping the needle within the skin itself.

In the late cases of subluxation and fracture of coccyx also, the above procedure can be adopted. However, in early cases and in acute coccydodynia, injection of long-acting local anesthetic has been proved to be of more value.

Fibro-fatty Nodules (Figure 14.3B)

These have been blamed for producing symptoms akin to sciatic radiculitis (pseudosciatica). They usually lie in about upper sacroiliac zones where they can be rolled under the fingers. Nodules are frequently tender and may trigger the pain down along the course of sciatic nerve. These nodules should be infiltrated into and around by direct approach over it. Depending upon the relief obtained, the corticosteroid cocktail may be repeated at two weekly intervals.

INFILTRATION INTO AND AROUND SCIATIC NERVE

For intractable sciatic radicular pain, injection of local anesthetic with or without the corticosteroid, in and around the sciatic nerve in its course through the lower buttock or upper thigh can be helpful.

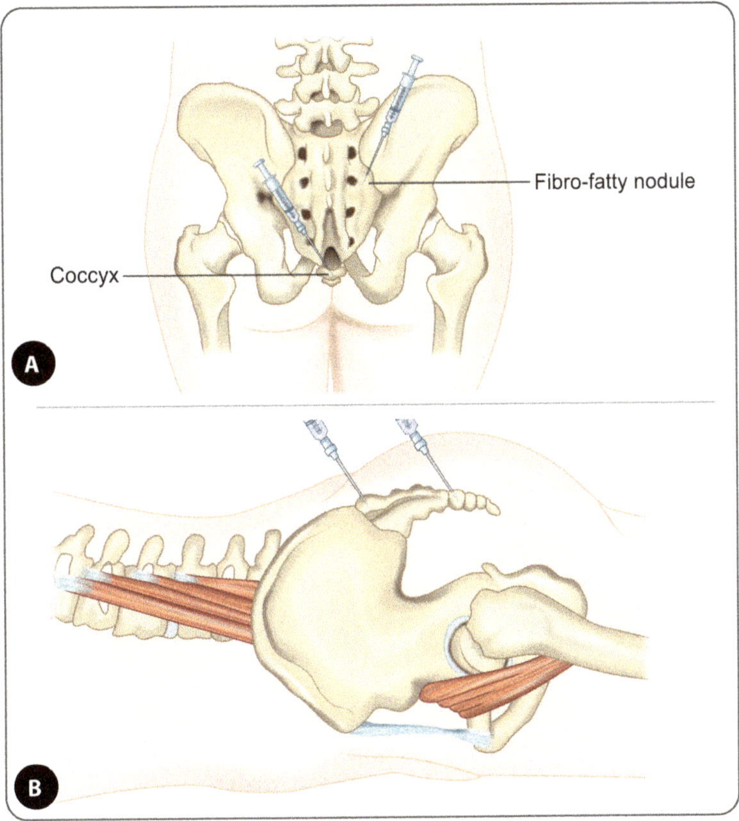

FIGS. 14.3A AND B: Injection for: Coccydodynia, fibro-fatty nodule: (A) Back view, (B) Side view.

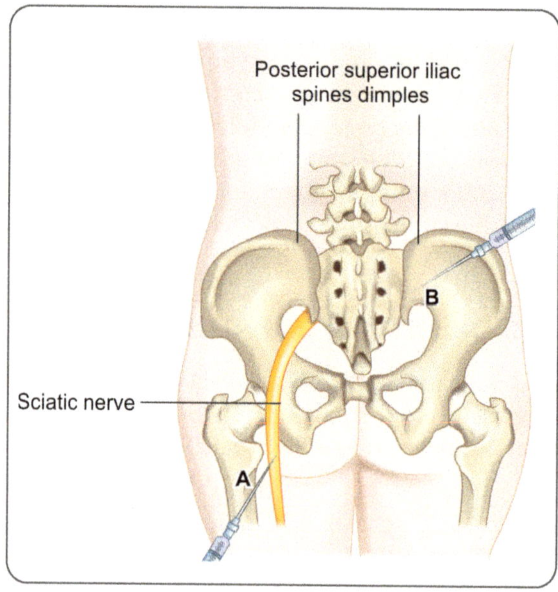

FIGS. 14.4A AND B: (A) Approach to sciatic nerve (in and around); (B) Approach to sacroiliac joint.

Method (Figure 14.4)

Along the anatomical course of sciatic nerve, at about the center of lower gluteal fold, pressing against the femur the sciatic nerve can be rolled or a tender course of the nerve can be delineated except in fatty patients. Injection should be given directly through a long thin slender needle along the tender course at any convenient point in and around sciatic nerve.

OLD PELVIC FRACTURE

At times, patients do complain of discomfort and a varying amount of persistent pain in and around the fractured pelvis area, especially the rami. The affected area, if palpably tender, may be infiltrated with corticosteroid cocktail at weekly intervals three to seven sittings.

RECURRENT FIBROSITIS

In recurrent fibrositis, either at the root of the neck or anywhere in the span of lumbosacral fascia, local injection of corticosteroid cocktail often gives a considerable relief.

RHEUMATOID SPONDYLITIS

Corticosteroid injection into sacroiliac joint gives symptomatic relief in this condition.

SACROILIAC JOINT

Indications

- Sacroiliac strains and sprains
- Rheumatoid arthritis
- Ankylosing spondylitis
- Unexplained tenderness in the region of sacroiliac.

Method (Figure 14.4)

The patient lies prone or on the side. Sacroiliac joints fortunately are represented superficially by obvious dimples. These dimples are more or less superficial to posterior superior iliac spine and adjoining part of upper sacroiliac joint. These can be easily seen and felt even in obese individuals. The fingertip passing down and posteriorly with slight outer inclination over the posterior part of the iliac crest can easily locate the comparatively rough posterior margin of the joint. Needle should be pushed directly into the joint. Occasionally, the fibro-fatty nodules (responsible for pseudosciatica like condition) also lie in this region. These nodules can also be adequately infiltrated by direct 'touch-feel-inject' technique. In sacral region, indications may be akin to those of the lower spine. In conditions, like fibrotic nodule, fibrofascitis, degenerative conditions, painful spasm in ankylosing spondylitis, rheumatoid arthritis and discitis, corticosteroid cocktail injection may have a role, but our experience in this region has been limited.

CHAPTER 15

Facial Region

"You hesitate to stab me with a word, and know not—silence is the sharper sword."

—Samuel Johnson

CHAPTER OUTLINE

- Oral cavity

In **atrophic rhinitis** and **recurrent allergic rhinitis**, corticosteroid infiltration has been found to give relief. This must be done under direct vision using very thin sharp needle working submucously.

ORAL CAVITY

Post-traumatic or post-infective facial contractures, if infiltrated with corticosteroid cocktail combined with gradual stretching may yield satisfactory results.

The **pale mucosal fibrosis** (a rare condition) produces gradual extra-articular ankylosis of the jaw. Since etiology is not exactly known, the recommended treatment has been empirical. Though difficult to prognosticate, repeated submucosal corticosteroid infiltration must be tried at bi-weekly intervals combined with gradual stretching of the jaws. Almost similar clinical condition is oral submucous fibrosis, a well-known clinical entity, has been seen in about 13% of general population—more in southern States of India. The exact cause is not known, however, prolonged use of chilly, betel nut, tobacco, alcohol, *Pan masala* and *Pan* has been the local irritating and causative factor (Jayavelu and Sambandan 2012). This condition was known even in Sushruta's period (600 BC) when it was called 'vidari.' The clinical features are according to the progress of disease right from blanching of oral mucosa without or with burning sensation, dryness of mouth, vesicles or ulcers in the mouth, decreasing of range of opening of mouth and protrusion of tongue. Jayavelu and Sambandan observed marked improvement in this condition with combined therapy with nutritional and iron supplements along with intralesional injection of hyaluronidase, dexamethasone, and placentrex and local application of anesthetic topical gel and **triamcinolone acetonide 0.1%**.

In the facial region, temporomandibular joint has been a frequent site for corticosteroid injection. Common indications are:

1. Fibrous ankylosis of jaw (following rheumatoid, trauma, subdued infection, idiopathic and degenerative arthrosis).
2. **Recurrent subluxation of the joint**.
3. **Snapping joint syndrome**.
4. **Postoperative ankylosis of jaw**.
5. Nonspecific synovitis.

Method (Figure 15.1)

It is better to inject with the patient lying with face turned to opposite side. However, it can also be done in sitting position with head supported on the back of chair. The patient lies down, and face is turned to opposite side as far as possible. Place the fingertip just in front and a little above the tragus, ask the patient to open and close the mouth frequently. One will be able to feel a gap running anteroposteriorly. While the patient is opening and closing the mouth, judge the position in which the gap is felt maximum. Ask the patient to keep the mouth open to that extent. If he/she is not cooperative, put a block in the mouth to maintain that position. Through the localized

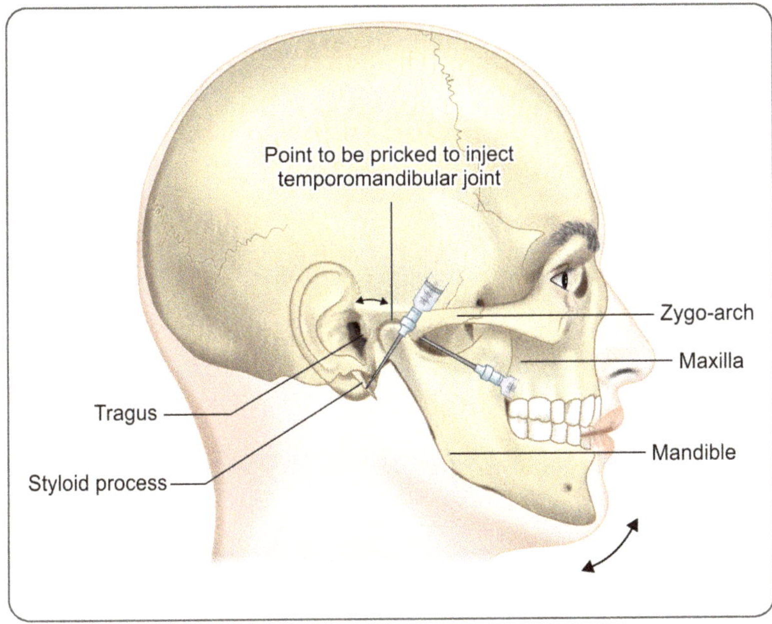

FIG. 15.1: Point to approach—temporomandibular joint.

gap, push the thin needle toward midline with slight downward inclination. If it is properly negotiated, loss of resistance will be felt. Repeatedly, confirm by aspiration, for avoiding injury to any vessel, e.g., internal maxillary. Inject a little local anesthetic and look for any effect in the distribution of facial nerve. At times, any of the branches may be injected, which should be avoided. However, if it happens, its effect will automatically dwindle off within 1-2 hours. Inject the corticosteroid cocktail into the joint. In bilateral cases, the same process can be repeated on contralateral side in the same sitting. Never try to puncture through oral cavity which is dirty, containing numerous organisms.

CHAPTER 16

Joints Around the Clavice

"Every time you tear a leaf off a calendar, you present a new place for new ideas and progress."

—Charles Kettering

CHAPTER OUTLINE

- Method

In painful chronic arthritis conditions, acromioclavicular joints are also involved. They may require corticosteroid injection as in other sites. Besides, traumatic synovitis, arthritis can also be the indications.

METHOD

Sternoclavicular Joint (Figure 16.1A)

The patient lies supine with a sandbag beneath the neck. Pass the finger medially along the upper border of clavicle. It will terminate into a bony projection. Just medial to it, a very narrow slit can be felt. Push the needle from superoanterior point of the slit, directly down with little posterior and outwards inclination and infiltrate into the joint. One should avoid going deep lest major vessels may come in the way.

Acromioclavicular Joint (Figure 16.1B)

The patient lies supine with scapular region supported on a sandbag. Follow the outer end of clavicle which ends in anterosuperior projection. Just outside it, a very narrow gap can be felt. Push the needle directly into the gap with posterior and a little downward inclination from superolateral to inferomedial direction. You are in the joint.

The nonspecific painful conditions with or without swelling of xiphisternum and/or costochondral junction can also be treated by local injection of corticosteroid cocktail with varying success. The technique will be more or less one of 'touching, feeling and injecting' the most tendor area.

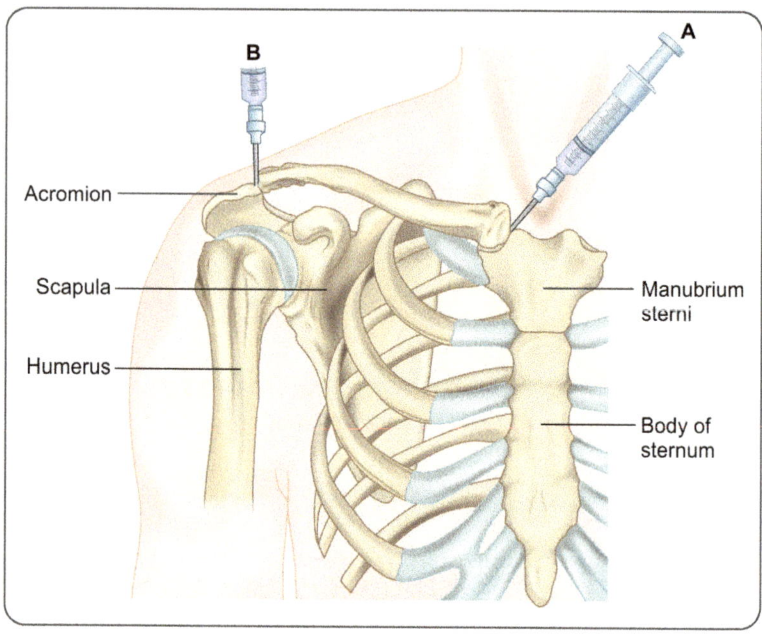

FIGS. 16.1A AND B: Injection into: (A) Sternoclavicular joint; (B) Acromioclavicular joint.

CHAPTER 17

Occipital Region

"He, who has not christmas in his heart, will never find it under a tree."

—Roy L Smith

CHAPTER OUTLINE

- Trigeminal neuralgia

In the occipital region there are not many indications for corticosteroid injection. The tender fibrotic nodules usually encountered in pressure area or in course of supranuchal line can be treated by corticosteroid injection. Posterior auricular nerve in **Hansen's pathology**, presenting with thickened nodule may be infiltrated with corticosteroid cocktail. In the scalp for localized alopecia, keratitis and leukoderma, local infiltration of corticosteroid has been tried with varying results.

Ophthalmic indications of corticosteroid are limited. However, in nonspecific keratitis, ocular opacity, fibrotic infiltration of sclera and at times viral ocular palsy, corticosteroid has been used.

In the facial region, keloids of any region, papillary warts, contact dermatitis and chronic herpetic eruptions may be the indications for corticosteroid injection depending on the clinician's choice.

In **Bell's palsy**, theoretically, injection of corticosteroids in and around the stylomastoid foramen may have a local anti-inflammatory action.

Method: The patient lies on the side. In posterior digastric fossa just behind the neck of mandible, the needle can be pushed, directed medially with downward and posterior inclination taking all possible care of avoiding carotid vessels (by pulsation). Usually, the needle tip, if negotiated gradually, hits the bony margin. Pull the needle a little and infiltrate the cocktail.

In **trigeminal neuralgia,** corticosteroid cocktail may give symptomatic relief and sometimes lasting relief to the patients.

Method (Figure 17.1): Feel the zygomatic notch, and insert the needle 1 cm below it. Advance the tip upwards, backwards and inwards to about 5 cm depth. As the needle tip touches the third division of the trigeminal nerve,

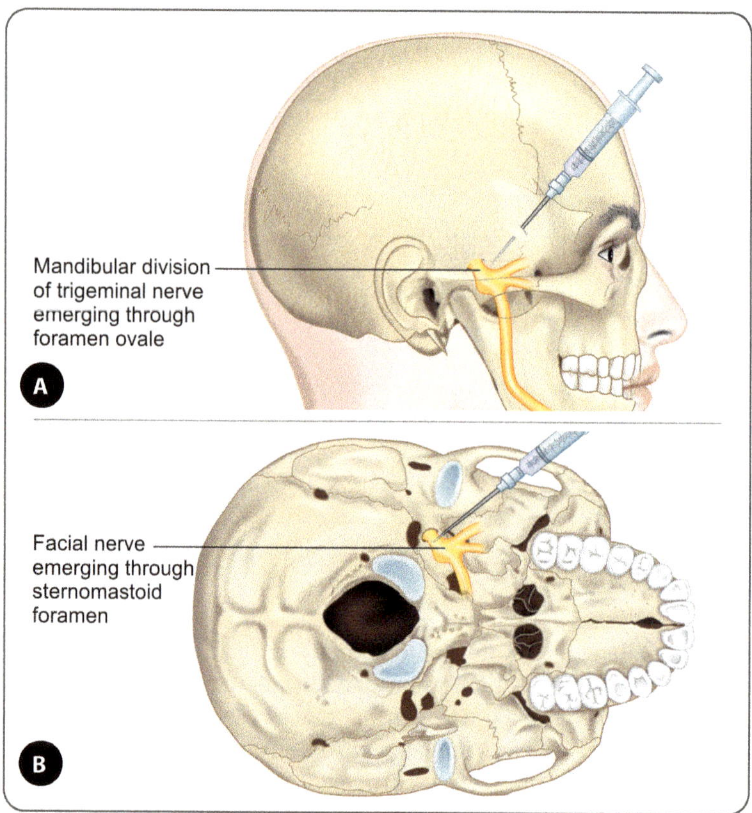

FIGS. 17.1A AND B: Method of injecting for trigeminal neuralgia. (A) The position of injecting needle is shown in ralation to the mandibular division of trigeminal nerve on the lateral side of face. (B) The position of needle is shown in relation to the facial nerve on the base of skull. In trigeminal neuralgia, corticosteroid acetate cocktail may give symptomatic relief and some times lasting relief to the patients.

the patient experiences severe pain. Local anesthetic should be injected immediately. The needle point is further advanced. When some resistance is felt, the tip is in the vicinity of the trigeminal ganglion. The corticosteroid cocktail or 4 mL of absolute alcohol may be injected slowly watching for any side effect simultaneously.

It is difficult to predict the lasting effects of the injection. However, if two consecutive injections are not markedly helpful, it is worthwhile going for resection of the sensory root in the middle cranial fossa.

TRIGEMINAL NEURALGIA

Trigeminal neuralgia, a benign disease, may be defined as short, sharp, lancinating paroxysmal unilateral pain in the area of trigeminal nerve distribution.

The disease mainly affects the elderly age group with more incidence in females, however, about 10% of patients are below 40 years of age.

Right side has been seen to be most affected. Usually, the pain appears paroxysmally lasting for a few seconds with free periods in between the attacks. As the disease advances, the number of attacks increases and the free periods become gradually shorter. Ultimately, the pain becomes continuous and agonising which even may push the patient to suicidal point. Any movement of jaws (like chewing, talking, etc.), washing of face, exposure to cold wind, etc., precipitates the shooting pain. Usually, a trigger spot develops in the face region, over which even a gentle touch initiates the sudden sharp shooting trigeminal pain.

Etiology

The exact cause is not known. However, **vascular compression** (usually by superior cerebellar artery or anterior inferior cerebellar artery) at the **TREZ** (**T**rigeminal **R**oot **E**ntry **Z**one) has been blamed for this pain. With the advancing age the arteries become sclerotic and stiff which can cause more pressure.

Other Probable Causes

Idiopathic demyelination of the nerve may result in ephaptic transmission of impulses (i.e., **"cross talking" of the axons** where in ordinary touch sensation is felt as pain sensation).

In **multiple sclerosis**, sometimes trigeminal pain precipitates.

Tumors in cerebellopontine angle (e.g., **meningioma, acoustic neuroma, epidermoid**) may lead to **trigeminal neuralgia**.

Diagnosis is mainly on typical history. The patient may precipitate the pain by finding the trigger zone. Objective sensory loss or motor involvement is mainly due to some intracranial organic lesion.

CT scan or MRI is usually normal in idiopathic trigeminal neuralgia; however, only cerebellopontine angle tumor or other organic lesions can be delineated by CT scan or MRI.

Trigeminal neuralgia can be confused with toothache (where pain is continuous), **sphenopalantine neuralgia**, atypical facial pain, diabetic cranial neuropathy, glaucoma, etc.

Management is medical or surgical—limited invasion; or major intracranial operations, e.g., retromastoid craniotomy and macrovascular decompression. Various medicines (such as carbamazepine phenytoin, baclofen, clonazepam, gabapentin, etc.) have been tried with varied degree of success for varied period.

For the refractory patients, other options are:
- **Corticosteroid cocktail injections**
- Peripheral neurectomy

- Rhizolysis with glycerol or radiofrequency lesions, which results in severe dysesthetic pain, which may be sometimes even more worse for the patient
- Percutaneous **trigeminal ganglion balloon compression (PTBC)**, which is at present perhaps the best choice in percutaneous treatment. Here, under general anesthesia, a wide-bore needle is passed into the foramen ovale. A balloon catheter is introduced into the **Meckel's cave**. The balloon is inflated to compress over the preganglionic and ganglionic fibres, which relieves the pain.

It provides long-lasting relief and is suitable for the elderly patients (even complicated with, diabetes, hypertension, coronary artery compromised conditions).

In resistant cases or cases with organic lesions major open-skull surgical operations (e.g., **retromastoid craniectomy** and **macrovascular decompression**) may be required.

CHAPTER 18

Complications of Intra-articular Injections

"The only point in listing some of the possible complications is to expect them, watch for them and deal with them promptly when they arise."

—**SP**

CHAPTER OUTLINE

- Complications due to lack of aseptic procedure
- Management of infection
- Complications due to error on the part of clinicians
- Corticosteroids can produce general complications
- Complications due to the drug
- Rebound phenomenon
- Delayed manifestations of infections

COMPLICATIONS DUE TO LACK OF ASEPTIC PROCEDURE

Mild-to-moderate, even severe infection (may be associated with features of bacteremia, pyemia, septicemia, even shock) may occur. Unfortunately, this is a common complication. This may even lead to persistent, incapacitating, chronic infection lingering on for years.

1. **Infective arthritis:** It is a major complication which is becoming less, thanks to proper antiseptic care and single-use equipment (syringe tray). It is being estimated at about 1 per 10,000, in Western advanced setups. But it still represents a fair number of the arthritis observed in medical practice. It manifests 24–36 hours after injection, by intense joint inflammation associated in 50% of cases with hyperthermia. Diagnosis rests on aspiration of joint, cytological examination (highly inflammatory fluid, very rich in altered polynuclear cells) and bacteriologic culture (*Staphylococcus aureus* in 50%). Patil SD et al. (2015) have reported a case of acute compartment syndrome of foot developed due to infection secondary to local hydrocortisone injection given to treat plantar fascitis.

How to know the onset of infection?

Usually, after 24 hours of injection, such patients start having increasing swelling and clear inflammatory features (rubor, calor, dolor, tumor, functio laesa), features of cellulitis, pitting edema, fluctuant accumulation in the joint, even bursting of the abscess and resultant sinus. Constitutional features may accompany to a variable extent, in the earlier phase.

2. **Acute post-infiltrative inflammation:** Mild local reactions may occur after injection. Microcrystalline arthritis induced by corticosteroids suspensions, i.e., the chemical synovitis in a reactive manifestation to the injected crystals may manifest in about 5% of the cases. Appearing as acute incident in the early hours following infection (cf-delayed manifestations in sepsis) expressed by a recrudescence of pain with moderate local inflammatory phenomena. The features disappear spontaneously in a few hours; however, local application of ice helps.
   Flushing of face may be seen in 10–15% of cases, mainly in women.
3. **Tendon ruptures:** Following repeated infiltrations of corticosteroids, rupture of the tendon is not unusual, especially in Achilles heel tendinitis. Intratendinous injection should be avoided as the tendon remains already fragile. The number of infiltrations should be limited in tenosynovitis and tendinitis of the shoulder and elbow.
4. **Destructive "steroid" arthropathy:** Repeated use of local corticosteroid may produce accelerated destruction of joints; whether due to deleterious action of corticosteroids on cartilage or cartilage overaction after relief of pain—exact cause is not known. However, if indicated for longer period, interval of prick should be prolonged.
5. **Local skin depigmentation.**
6. **Atrophy of cutaneous and subcutaneous tissues and fat atrophy may be seen at the site of injecting point:** Repeated infiltration and particularly those of fluorinated cortisone derivatives, (betamethasone, triamcinolone) can produce atrophy of skin and subcutaneous tissue. It has been especially seen in superficial tendinopathies (elbow, wrist, finger region). Hence, in such lesions, prednisolone acetate (3 injections) should be preferred.
7. **Intratendinous and intrabursal precipitate.**
8. **General effects of local corticosteroid therapy:** Though the therapeutic objective of local corticosteroid infiltration is to avoid the complication of general corticosteroid therapy, but prolonged local use (for months/years) can induce general side effects (osteoporosis, cataract, cortico-suprarenal insufficiency, probably, due to diffusion even of suspension).

MANAGEMENT OF INFECTION

1. **Prophylactic:** Even with very little doubt in aseptic procedure, it is rewarding to prescribe broad-range antibiotics for 6–7 days following the injection.

2. With the earliest features of inflammation, suspect the imminent severe infection and treat it on war-footing with:
   a. Rest to the part either by support or splintage or by traction, as applicable.
   b. Broad-range antibiotics, especially staphylococcal-oriented.
   c. Hot-moist fomentation, 3–4 times daily.
   d. Analgesics.
   e. Vitamin B complex and vitamin C.
3. If the features do not start subsiding within 24 hours, there is no harm in putting a wide-bore needle, aspirating the collection, washing the joint with normal saline and injecting antibiotic solution whatever available, pending the result of culture and sensitivity report of the aspirated material. Depending upon the response, the procedure may be repeated even daily combined with suitable antibiotics.
4. Watch the progress. If infection is organising, same procedure may be repeated and continued. If response is not favorable, no time should be lost in performing arthrotomy of the joint, thorough lavage and suitable antibiotic instillation.

   One has to bargain in such circumstances. The infected synovium is a constant source of infection which persists or recurs at intervals. Hence, whenever suspicion exists, synovectomy may be combined in the same sitting. The joint should be closed with continuous closed 'irrigation-suction drainage system,' i.e., with the inflowing tube, normal saline with suitable detergent and antibiotic solution is dropped into the joint and through the outflowing tube dirty fluid is drained out.
5. In late cases, with or without sinus, the treatment is the same as that of old septic infections of the joint or other sites. For the joint, ultimately, it may amount to excision-arthrodesis.
6. In very unfortunate circumstances, the infection may persist for pretty long time incapacitating the patient for variable periods. Sometimes the treating team and or the patient gets terribly annoyed of the persistent infection and then the patient asks for persistently and then one may consider to dispense with the affected part.

For general complications of pyogenic infection, i.e., bacteremia, pyemia, septicemia and shock, the treatment must be on war footing to avoid the hazardous outcome. Besides managing the local infection as above, the possible general complications must be carefully attended from the very beginning—such as:

1. Managing shock.
2. Fluid balance.
3. Suitable antibiotic cover.
4. Electrolyte balance.
5. Blood transfusion, if needed.
6. General build-up.
7. Maintaining kidney function.
8. Protein build-up.

COMPLICATIONS DUE TO ERROR ON THE PART OF CLINICIANS

1. Infections (vide supra).
2. Difficulty or error in selecting the point of injection: In such circumstances, not only the drug does not reach the desired point but it also initiates pain on a site which was hitherto painless.
3. Pushing the needle too deep, so that it strikes the articular cartilage or bony component: Instantaneously, the patient feels sharp pain. Subsequently, effusion may appear with increasing pain. Varying limitations of movements of the joint (spasmodic) may develop. This can be avoided by cautiously pushing the needle into the joint area. However, if it happens, reassurance, cold compress, analgesics and rest to the part for about two days usually provide marked relief.
4. Sometimes error has been noticed in the materials injected, which can produce complications.

CORTICOSTEROIDS CAN PRODUCE GENERAL COMPLICATIONS

- With triamcinolone hexacetonide (THA) injection, hot flushes and facial redness have been observed
- With methylprednisolone acetate (MPA) also, rarely may be local burning sensation, or rashes
- Intra-articular injection of bupivacaine and methylprednisolone, there may be anaphylaxis
- Repeated intra-articular corticosteroids may lead to local osteonecrosis and marrow fat-induced synovitis
- Methylprednisolone acetate has been observed to provide better response initially for a few weeks.

COMPLICATIONS DUE TO THE DRUG

As such, anaphylactic reaction and other untoward reactions have been very rarely reported. Hydrocortisone acetate, itself being of corticosteroid group, is least likely to produce reaction as far as the drug is concerned. Perhaps, reactions noted after hydrocortisone acetate injection might be due to the local anesthetic used. However, we had occasions to note peculiar reactive changes following intra-articular hydrocortisone acetate injection. Patients started complaining of piercing pain in the joint which showed some amelioration following gentle movement of the joint. Again, after about 2 hours, they had severe pain in the joint with a sense of exhaustion in the whole body. Thence, a swelling about an inch in diameter appeared on contralateral infrapatellar fossa of the same knee. This was evidenced on both knees in one case where both were injected in the same sitting.

General condition of the patients was perfectly all right. They required a good amount of sedative for relief of pain. Such conditions persisted for 18–20 hours. Again, we are not able to say whether it was due to hydrocortisone acetate or local anesthetic. Sometimes, the patient complains of heaviness in the joint which persists for a day. Whether it is an effect of local prick or due to injected volume of the drug, could not be ascertained. However, this is not a regular phenomenon.

REBOUND PHENOMENON

It has been noticed that very occasionally the patient gets marked relief of symptoms following even the first prick, but the symptoms reappear with greater magnitude even when the treatment line remains exactly the same and with no features of inflammation. These symptoms do persist for very long periods. No suitable explanation for this bizarre manifestation can be offered.

DELAYED MANIFESTATIONS OF INFECTIONS

Very rarely, we had the occasion of seeing the patients with delayed infection in whom injection was given elsewhere months or years back. The patient presented with subdued features of septic arthritis and we had diagnosed as a case of nonspecific or subacute pyogenic arthritis. When arthrotomy was done, chalky white deposits of previously injected hydrocortisone acetate were noticed, round about which the chronic infiltrative reactive features were also observed.

On histopathological examination, the features of chronic pyogenic arthritis in two cases and chronic nonspecific arthritis in one case were reported. Culture were sterile in all the three cases.

CHAPTER 19

Role of Botulinum Toxin Type A Injection in Spastics and Other Indications

"Success is most often achieved by those who don't know that failure is inevitable."

—Coco Chanel

CHAPTER OUTLINE

- Botulinum toxin type A
- Mode of working of botulinum toxin type A (BT-A—BOTOX)

Spasticity results due to insult, injury or damage to either the brain or spinal cord or both [central nervous system (CNS)], e.g., cerebral palsy, cerebrovascular accidents, multiple sclerosis, spinal cord injury. Spasticity may be generalized affecting large part of body or it may affect small area such as wrist, hand, ankle (focal spasticity). The severity of spasticity may vary ranging from mild muscle stiffness to severe painful uncontrollable muscle spasm which can affect sitting in a chair or even lying in bed and can make moving from one place or position to another very difficult. Spasticity is almost always a life-long problem. If left neglected, it gradually worsens and ends in contractures.

The most important treatment of spasticity is regular physical therapy and relaxing and stretching exercises. Proper treatment of spasticity depends upon the pattern and degree of spasticity. If there is a large area affected by spasticity, oral medication or intrathecal medication may be required. If a relatively small area is affected local injection of drugs like phenol or botulinum toxin type A (BT-A available as **BOTOX or BOTOGenie**) may be given to weaken or paralyse specific overactive muscles. Severe spasticity which cannot be effectively treated with drugs or injections may require surgery. However, physiotherapy and occupational therapy must be continued along with.

Ethyl alcohol and BT-A injections are being used for treating spastic cerebral palsy and becoming popular due to, their localized effects, minimal systemic side effect, ease of application and obviously improved functional outcome of patients.

Comparative improvement in spasticity has been observed with both ethyl alcohol and BT-A. Significant improvement of gastrocnemius muscle power occurs after use of both, however, more with BT-A.

BOTULINUM TOXIN TYPE A

Botulinum toxin type A is a natural purified protein, whose active ingredient is BT-A and is extracted from bacteria under controlled laboratory conditions.

MODE OF WORKING OF BOTULINUM TOXIN TYPE A (BT-A—BOTOX)

The electrochemical messages are transmitted from the higher center to the muscle through the nerves. At the nerve-endings acetylcholine is secreted which initiates the muscular contractions. If due to irratic or abnormal or asynchronus or excessive release of neuromuscular signals too much of acetylcholine is released at the neuromuscular junctions, it induces overactivity in muscular contractions leading to muscle spasm.

Once injected BT-A binds to the nerve terminal and blocks the release of acetylcholine relaxing overactive muscles. BT-A temporarily blocks the nerve's ability to release acetylcholine, and thus, greatly reduces or even stops muscle spasms which relieves the symptoms.

BT-A has been used since 1989 to treat several conditions presenting with spasticity, especially, in the face, e.g., in the management of **blepharospasm**, neck muscle spasm, etc. BT-A injections remove the frawn lines. The person looks less depressed and appears less angry after injection. In blepharospasm BT-A is given 0.1 mL or less just under the skin and into the muscles around the eye that cause the increased blinking. BT-A reduces both the strength and frequency of contraction of the eyelid muscles, and thus, improves the symptoms. The effect lasts for about 6 months after which injection should be repeated.

To get rid of fine creases, lines and wrinkle of face and other facial rejuvenation certain injectable treatment, such as use of fillers and paralytic agents, has been tried. Fillers are of several types such as:

- Autologous fat.
- Shelf fillers synthetic like Sculptra
- Animal derived fillers like collagen
- Hyaluronic acid fascian
- Human cadaveric tissue like AlloDerm or Cymetra.

These fillers fill up in and around the area of tissue deficiency. They work remarkably for a while, but these are not permanent solution, since the underlying muscle's action and other causes of the facial lines are not corrected. Further tissue rejection to implanted foreign body is also a problem, Botulinum toxin is commonly used as muscle paralytic agent. This is also a temporary solution to the underlying cause of facial lines, especially those between the eyebrows or the forehead. However, Botox (Botulinum A exotoxin) is a safe and effective treatment for relaxation of fascial lines and wrinkles. When injected into certain facial muscles, it relaxes these muscles, thus smoothening out the wrinkles. It lasts for 3–6 months. The treatment may be repeated for continuous effect.

In cerebral palsy children, excessive drooling (sialorrhea) can be reduced/checked by injecting BT-A into the salivary glands under USG/image guidance to block their function.

In the spastics, the appropriate indication of BT-A injection is in those where joints can be moved passively and where it is anticipated that weakening of the targeted muscles will not reduce the functional capacity. BT-A injection is almost the treatment of choice in very young children with gastrocnemius spasticity, recommended as a time-buying agent in children who are not suitable for surgery. Besides its use in spastics (mainly cerebral palsy), BT-A is being used in several medical specialities, e.g., by orthopedicians, dermatologists (cosmetic enhancement of face), neurologists, physichiatrists, proctologists, rehabilitationists, gastroenterologists, etc. Xu et al. (2015) have used BT-A injection combined with cast immobilization for treating recurrent peroneal spastic flatfoot without bone coalitions.

BT-A is injected in the prior-selected muscles which are having spasm with or without pain. The target muscles are identified by using electrical stimulation with the probe attached to the needle passed into the suspected muscle. After confirming the targeted muscle BT-A is injected into that muscle/s. Small muscle should be injected at 1–2 sites, whereas the larger muscles may require 3–4 injections (sites). The effect of BT-A remains more or less confined to the injected muscle only in the area of 2–3 cm around the site of injection. The injection is like any other intramuscular injection or with little more discomfort. In apprehensive patients, local anesthetic cream or spray may be used. Since BT-A is a biological product, one cannot rule out the possibility of anaphylactic reaction. Hence, one should be ready to tackle it and epinephrine and respiratory support should be readily available.

The effect of BT-A injection usually starts after a few days with obvious beneficial effect by 2 weeks. The beneficial effect lasts for about 3–4 months, after which muscle starts returning to its pre-injection condition. Proper physiotherapy must be continued while the effect of BT-A injection is fully available. BT-A injection can be continued as long as the condition responds to the treatment and does not have any serious allergic reactions or other side effects. However, long-term usage of BT-A can lead to resistance in a patient due to development of antibodies.

There are no serious complications of BT-A injections. Locally, there may be variable pain, tenderness and bruising. Rarely, there may be symptoms such as, joint pain, headache, skin rashes, nausea, swelling, redness, bruising, bleeding, dizziness, pruritis, muscle-stiffness, reduced coordination, excessive inactivation of nearby muscles if dose is more. It is not like other complications, however cost factor matters, especially in the management of cerebral palsy children. This may be tackled as follows. The use of BT-A has increased in plastic surgical clinics for cosmetic enhancements (for the persons who can afford well). The volume of injections is less in the face. However, the left over toxin in the vial should not be thrown, since it can be used in spastic muscles of cerebral palsy children, and thus, overall cost is reduced. The toxin refrigerated at +4°C or refrozen at -20°C does not loose its potency and can be effectively used as the fresh reconstituted BT-A (Botox)-(Sloop et al. 1997), except for the possibility of bacterial contamination. On overall consideration, BT-A treatment is costly and unless subsidized by the government or some philanthropic body or NGOs, it may not be viable at least for cerebral palsy patients.

There is hardly any systemic spread of the toxin. Even one vial of (100 units) BT-A is below the systemic toxicity of human beings weighing 6 kg or more. It has been assumed that 3,000 units of BT-A would be lethal in the human (Chutorian and Root 1994).

CHAPTER 20

Cell Therapy Transplantation of Bone Marrow Cells

"A brave leader will have a 'never-say-never' attitude because of his strong vision and passion."

—Dr APJ Abdul Kalam

CHAPTER OUTLINE

- Stem cell
- Stem cells: A preliminary look
- Cell therapy
- Transplantation of bone marrow cells

STEM CELL

The concept of "Regenerative Medicine" was introduced by Leland Kaiser in 1992, who forecasted that "a new branch of medicine will develop that attempts to change the course of chronic diseases and in many instances will regenerate the tired and failing organ systems" (Kaisar LR 1992).

Scientists since then, are engaged to develop cell-based approaches to regenerate damaged tissues or even substitute whole organ. Stem cell are of particular interest in regenerating medicine. They inherit several unique characteristics that distinguish from other cell types. However, the ideal carrier for the stem cells remains controversial. The application of stem cells in regenerative medicine for orthopedic indication is being variously studied both in experimental animals and clinical possible indications. Shape with specialized function, such as heart, skin or nerve cells (Anderson et al. 2001). Broadly stem cells can be differentiated into two types: (i) Totipotent cells, which can form any tissue, e.g., fertilized egg or zygote; (ii) Pluripotent cells, which have less differentiating capacity, e.g., embryonic stem cells; (iii) Multipotent cells which are capable to differentiate into one particular ceil type only, e.g., bone marrow stromal or mesenchymal stem cells.

STEM CELLS: A PRELIMINARY LOOK

A stem cell is an immature undifferentiated cell which has the capability of producing identical daughter cell(s). After differentiation the cell becomes capable to form mesenchymal stem cells (MSCs) it has been proved to have enormous potential in the field of management of degenerative diseases related to neuronal, cardiac and bony tissues of the human body. The pioneering work of Friedenstein et al. in mid sixties (1966, 1968, 1970) opened the vista of evidence for the potentiality of the stem cells, present in the bone marrow, to produce nonhematopoietic progeny. These cells in bone marrow are of mesenchymal origin (hence, they are called Mesenchymal stromal/stem cells-MSCs), which are the plastic adherent young cells and are capable of forming clonal fibroblast colony (CFU-f).

Friedenstein et al. also suggested the basic technique of isolating BM-MSCs by only bone marrow with suitable medium on the disc. The supernatant portion (nonhematopoietic adhered cells) is discarded after 24 hours, and the adherent cells are left back.

The multipotent characters of MSCs have been proved and they can differentiate into osteoblasts, chondroblasts and adipocytes. They can rescue or repair the injured and degenerating cells. These cells have capacity of expressions of immunomodulatory and tropical factors. These cells have exhibited immense potential in repair and regeneration.

Source of Stem Cells

There are many sources of stem cells which can be used for tissue repair and regeneration, few examples:

1. **Embryonic stem cells**, which are pluripotent and can self-replicate. They are isolated from the inner cell mass of blastocyst. These stem cells have potential for bone formation in humans. They represent the only cell type, which has the ability to renew itself indefinitely and is truly pluripotent.
2. **Adult stem cell (ASC):** They have limited regeneration capacity and only for the tissues they reside in (big bone marrow, cornea, retina, liver, pancreas). ASC can replenish the cells of organ when they are lost due to injury or disease.
3. **Mesenchymal stem cells:** A type of adult stem cells—can be obtained by bone marrow, periosteum, skin, fat. These cells are multipotent and differentiate into chondrocyte, osteoblast, myoblast, etc. They can be used to treat osteogenesis imperfecta.

Mechanisms of action of stem cells are by:

1. Differentiation into cell types, such as: neuronal differentiation, cardiac differentiation, osteogenic differentiation.
2. Immunomodulatory effects
3. Paracrine mechanism (of action of MSCs)
4. Tissue engineering, such as:
   - Bone tissue engineering
   - Cardiac tissue engineering.

The basis of tissue engineering is the stem cells. In tissue engineering, an optimum and appropriate environment is created which governs cellular process in vivo. The cells are directed to differentiate at the appropriate time, in the appropriate place and into the most appropriate phenotype.

Cell-based tissue engineering for musculoskeletal tissue repair regeneration holds great promise for the future, however, several issues concerning their subject remain still unanswered like legislation, ethical issues, overall success, cost, etc.

R1. To promote regeneration of hyaline cartilage in the chondral defects due to trauma and degeneration. Ultimately the regeneration of cartilage gets completely integrated with the surrounding cartilage and underlying bone: The cultured mesenchymal stem cells has been used to repair chondral defects in advanced osteochondritis dissecans.

R2. Fetal CNS tissue grafting is being experimented in rats and cats with severe cord injuries with initial encouraging results (Reier PJ 2004).

R3 and R4. Bone tissue engineering using mesenchymal stem cells, has shown a new technique with good promise to fill-up a good-sized bone defects, albeit the work is in advanced animal experiment stage.

R5. In animal (rabbits) experiments it was found that ACL reconstructions coated with stem cells resulted in healing by formation of intervening zone of cartilage resembling the chondral enthesis of normal ACL insertions and it had better strength and stiffness (Lim JK et al. 2004).

R6. Injection of genetically engineered mesenchymal stem cells into the paravertebral muscles in experimental murine model has lead to spinal fusion (Hasharoni et al. 2005).

R7. In children of osteogenesis imperfecta, the transplant of allogenic bone marrow, after ablation of their own bone marrow has shown significant improvement in the amount and quality of bone formation, which indicates the capability of mesenchymal cells in the graft of generate osteoblasts which can synthesize normal bone.

Stem cell transplantation is a novel and promising treatment for patients with moderate-to-severe cerebral palsy.

The study conducted by Chen et al. (2013) advocated an intraspinal infusion of autologous mesenchymal stem cells—derived neural stem cell for treating moderate-to-severe cerebral palsy patients. They observed optimal improvement in motor function, but not in language quotient just in 3 months after transplantation. However, rehabilitation treatments were also continued simultaneously. Several types of stem cells may be used in the treatment of cerebral palsy; such as human to embryonic neural stem cells, olfactory ensheathing cells are difficult to apply in clinical practice due to potential immunological rejection of xenogeneic cells, ethical arguments, high risk of transplantation within brain and difficulty of reported transplantations (Carroll JE, Mays RW 2011).

Uses of Stem Cell Therapy

Due to insufficient knowledge about the long-term effect and stability of the implanted stem cells into the repaired tissues and lack of potency of mesenchymal stem cells about their differentiation into other lineages, it has not been possible to exploit properly the uses of stem cell therapy.

As on today stem cell play important role in orthopedic regenerative medicine, as has been evidenced in animal research in the field of bone, tendon and cartilage repair, however, data about tendon repair is limited to animal studies.

At present great hope is set on role of stem cell in regenerative medicine in almost all medical fields.

Mesenchymal stem cells have been observed to be most useful as they have shown good differentiation potential toward cartilage, tendon and bone cells. Mesenchymal stem cells have the ability to migrate chemotactically to tissues showing inflammation and injury (Wang et al. 2002). The MSCs have potential to rebuild injured tissues and they also secrete growth factors which enhance tissue regeneration. Though MSC has shown promising results in animal experiments, clinical data are not yet available to authenticate for regular application of tendon repair.

In treatment of osteochondral lesions, all applications for clinical use are based on very small case series. The MSC application technique was adopted from clinical experience of autologous chondrocyte transplantation (fibrin, collagen gel, periosteal flap)—(Schmitt et al. 2012).

In bone the main focus of regenerative medicine has been on atrophic nonunion and replacement of lost bone tissue—as in severe trauma, gross infection, or after tumor destruction or excision.

IN ORTHOPEDIC PRACTICE, stem cell therapy has been used for:

1. Cartilage repair.
2. Spinal cord regeneration.
3. Tendon repair.
4. Treatment of osteochondral lesions.
5. Augmentation of ACL repair/reconstruction.
6. Atrophic pseudoarthrosis.
7. Osteogenesis imperfecta
8. Muscular dystrophies
9. Tendon and ligament repair
10. Intervertebral disc degeneration
11. Osteonecrosis of femoral head
12. Nonunion in long bones, e.g., tibial delayed or nonunion.

CELL THERAPY

In cell therapy cellular material is injected into a patient with an aim to replace the diseased or dysfunctional cells by healthy living cells.

Cell therapy is of two types:

1. Autologous cell therapy in which patient's own cells are injected.
2. Allogeneic cell therapy in which, universal cell therapies are carried out using donor cell.

In the process of cell therapy—first cells are harvested, then cells are put for cell culture, and finally the desired cells are implanted into the damaged tissue or damaged organ.

Benefits of Cell Therapy

- It is a targeted personalized cell therapy.
- It accelerates bone healing.
- It helps three-dimensional bone regeneration.
- It helps complete relief from pain.
- Progression of the disease is ceased.
- New blood supply is initiated, which further supports bone growth.

On the whole it helps in leading active normal life. With cartilage cell therapy, the benefits occurred are:

- It functions as personalized cell therapy.
- It initiates regeneration of hyaline like cartilage.
- It is minimally invasive procedure.
- It ceases progression of osteoarthritis.
- It completely restores the range of motion of the joint. Gradually it helps the patient to lead a normal life including the sports activities, e.g., the use of fibrin matrix mixed gel-type autologous chondrocyte implantation in the treatment for osteochondral lesions of the talus. Gel type ACL using autologous chondrocytes of the cuboid surface of the calcaneus was effective for improving talar cartilage defects was relatively easy to perform and did not induce morbidity at the donor site. (Lee et al. 2013).

TRANSPLANTATION OF BONE MARROW CELLS

(Based on medieval literature of pharma company SHIELD.) The success on bone marrow transplant or organ transplant could not be earlier successful because of the concept of presence of a biological force "the so-called transplantation antigen, which in human is named as human leukocyte antigens (HLA): This concept was suggested by Nobel Laureate Alexis Carrel (1912). The HLA antigens on the cell surface of transplanted organs are recognized by the recipient's immune defence as foreign and immunologically active cells try to reject the graft. Following transplantation of immunologically active cells—as in bone marrow transplantation—also the cells of the recipient are recognized as foreign, and the graft reacts against the cells of recipient in a way that can cause death. This reaction is called as the "graft-versus-host" reaction (GVH) and causes "graft-versus-host disease" (GVHD). The GVHD becomes the obstacle to the success of organ and cells transplant. However, in 1990 joint Nobel laureates in physiology and medicine Joseph E Murray and E Donnall Thomas opened the way for transplantation.

The discovery, that ionizing irradiation and cytotoxic drugs inhibit cell proliferation, made it possible to suppress the activity of the immune cells during transplantation, it was Joseph E Murray who showed that total body irradiation diminished the risk of rejection of the transplanted organ, Later he could show that a still better effect was obtained with the cytotoxic drug azathioprine. E Donnall Thomas on the other hand, managed to diminish the 'graft-versus-host, reaction by using another cytotoxic drug methotrexate. Thereby the way was opened for transplantation of the bone marrow cells.

CHAPTER 21

Acupuncture

"All things are possible until they are proven impossible."

—Pearl S Buck

CHAPTER OUTLINE

- Mode of working of acupuncture
- Acupuncture in low back pain
- Complications of acupuncture
- Acupuncture in arthritis
- Acupuncture in painful shoulder syndromes
- Acupressure
- Moxibustion

As written by Dr R Sharma (2012), the unknown clinicians worked constantly about 5,000 years to find out the means and way to alleviate the painful human ailments. Basing on their constant/continuous research for more than several hundred years, they located about 900 points in the body, pressing over which person can get rid of different complaints/diseases.

It is assumed that the discovering of principles and practice of Acupressure was done in India and from here, this science reached to China through Buddhists monks and travellers, where regular research works are being carried out. In due course, this system of treatment bifurcated in two systems: Acupressure and Acupuncture.

The Chinese have been claiming the immense role of acupuncture and moxibustion for managing several intractable maladies. Overall perusal indicates that in orthopedic arena this Chinese practice has only limited role. Once the bone is grossly involved, the outcome appears limited. However, on face value, acupuncture has been claimed to have symptomatic relief. Su Wen and Ling Shu tried to explain the basic principles of action of acupunctures as to balance the tissue activities, i.e., in case of **'Xu' (deficient activity)**, apply the **'Bu' (reinforcing method)**; and in case of **'Shi' (excessive activity)**, apply the **'Xie' (reducing method)**.

The mode of working of acupuncture is not that clear. Research is being conducted to investigate the biological mechanisms and pathways of acupuncture. The traditional chinese medicine uses acupuncture meridian theory which relates to the neurovascular tissue planes in the body. The acupuncture has a somatosensory stimulating effect leading to the release of endogenous opioids. The research has shown that acupuncture produces electrophysiologic changes in the nervous system leading to the release of neurotransmitters, neuropeptides and the body functions regulating hormones, due to the effect of acupuncture on the pituitary gland, autonomic nervous system and the brain as a whole. Despite several experimental and human studies concerning acupuncture, there is lack of consensus over explaining the mechanism of action, definite indications, number and locations of needle placements, efficacy of acupuncture points versus other points, manual versus electrical stimulations, period of relief, etc.

As an advancement, nowadays acupuncturists also use nonmeridian points and trigger points (tender sites in the most painful area). The needle may be stimulated, manually or electrically. To avoid infection stainless steel sterile disposable needles are being used.

The fact that the acupuncture analgesia may be mediated through the humoral factors, such as endogenous opioid peptides, has been gaining ground on the basis of recent experimental findings. Low-frequency electropuncture may be mediated in part by beta-endorphins while high frequency electroacupuncture may act through the serotonergic-enkephalinergic system.

As a method of substitute or synergism to hydrocortisone acetate injection into the joints or soft tissues (as discussed in previous chapters), the acupuncture system has some role in low backache, chronic nonspecific arthritis, painful shoulder syndrome, tennis elbow or allied conditions at elbow, **De Quervain's** disease and chronic sprain of lower extremities, especially the ankles. In these conditions too, once gross osteoarticular changes have occurred, the effect of this treatment is not very encouraging. So long as the explanation of the symptoms lies in and around the soft tissues, acupuncture can be an effective alternative tool in the hands of clinicians, especially when the available routine methods have proved ineffective. However, this is a job of an expert and must not be practised by clinicians unless prior practical course has been undergone.

ACUPUNCTURE IN LOW BACK PAIN

Acupuncture may be more effective in reducing the pain in short-term, but its effect is doubtful in the intermediate term in persons with chronic low back pain. As such acupuncture, along with no other treatment may be more effective in improving the chronic low back pain for initial 2–3 months. However, along with other treatments, like analgesics, NSAIDs, exercises, heat-therapy, mud packs, back care education, ergonomics and its improvements, etc., acupuncture may be more effective in improving the problems (pain and function) due to chronic low back pain.

COMPLICATIONS OF ACUPUNCTURE

Minor complications seen are local bleeding, hematoma, needling pain, vegetative symptoms, etc. There are very rare serious complications like infection (such as HIV, hepatitis, bacterial endocarditis), visceral trauma, such as pneumothorax.

ACUPUNCTURE IN ARTHRITIS

Commonly, rheumatic, rheumatoid and osteoarthritis conditions have been seen being treated in acupuncture clinics. During the acute stage of arthritis, treatment should be applied once every day. In the chronic conditions, treatment should be given every alternate day. The patient must be asked to undergo physiotherapy simultaneously for quicker recovery.

For low backache acupuncture and/or moxibustion have been frequently tried with, quite often, encouraging results. In acupuncture clinics, patients of sprained lumbar spine, rheumatoid spine, slipped discs, proliferative spondylitis, pelvic inflammatory diseases and even neoplastic conditions have been managed. However, the first three indications are suitable and in rest of the conditions acupuncture can be resorted to as an auxiliary treatment for symptomatic relief. For sprained spine strong stimulation and for muscular strains mild stimulation are given. Acupuncture and moxibustion can be applied simultaneously. Even electroneedling or cupping may also be applied. Treatment is done mainly through selected points, e.g., urinary bladder channels everyday or every other day retaining the needle for 15–20 minutes. After the pain is relieved, the local points are punctured.

ACUPUNCTURE IN PAINFUL SHOULDER SYNDROMES

Conditions like sprain, strain, peripheral nonspecific inflammation, supraspinatus tendinitis, subacromial bursitis, biceps tenosynovitis (tendinitis), have been managed by these methods. Fairly strong stimulations are given. Points are selected from the extremities. While manipulating the needle, the patient is asked to exercise the affected shoulder vigorously. Treatment may be given daily or on alternative day.

For tennis elbow, strong stimulations are given at local and distal points.

At the wrist and hand region, **De Quervain's disease**, trigger finger and tendon sheath ganglion have been treated by acupuncture with or without moxibustion. Medium to strong stimulation are given daily or every other day. However, corticosteroid injections, manipulations and surgical treatment have also been recommended as and when needed.

As posted by Samantha Powell on August 23rd, 2013, [http:///www.healthemi.com/acupuncturist-news-online/813-lungcancerli41v3]—Researchers concluded that acupuncture has been found to be effective in the management of pain in lung cancer with a sense of well-being. There is reduction of pain, nausea, nervousness, shortness of breadth, drowsiness and depression.

Chun-Hui Bao et al. have used moxibustion and acupuncture for the treatment of **Crohn's disease**, and have observed that this combined management is safe and effective for Crohn's disease.

ACUPRESSURE

Acupressure is a variant of Indian deep-massage and manipulation systems of *Prakriti Chikitsa* and *Ayurveda*. In China also this system is very popular. In acupressure, the treatment is imparted by putting pressure on specific points of human body for specific ailment. The principle of treatment is based on the integrated considerations of psychosoma, i.e., the physical anatomico-physiological body and associated psychological considerations.

The propagatists of acupressure suggest that the principle points controlling blood circulation, nerve distributions, nervous system control, endocrinal control and associated systems are situated in the central regions of palms and soles. Different pressure points control the different regions of body. When pressure is applied on any point, it triggers its controlling zone. If any area/zone/organ is unhealthy, its controlling point when pressed, induces pain.

Our body is made up of five basic elements—earth, fire, wind, water, space/sky—and these are regulated by some bioenergy (not clearly known). In any unhealthy/diseased condition, the balance of bioenergy control is disturbed and it may go astray. The proper pressure on the controlling point regulates the energy flow, and thus, improves or even cures the ailment.

Acupressure is supposed to increase the agility of body and flexibility of muscles, coordinated control of nervous system, sharpness of mind, function of endocrinal glands and overall functions of the internal organs of body.

The World Health Organization (WHO) has acknowledged the utility of acupressure and acupuncture medication system especially in the conditions such as sciatic radiculitis, cervical spondylosis, migraine, dyspepsia, sinusitis, gastritis, adhesive capsulitis (frozen shoulder) of shoulder, osteoarthritis, asthma, etc.

MOXIBUSTION

Moxibustion, based on the principle of thermal stimulation perhaps works as a counter-irritant and as a counter-physical stimulant.

Moxibustion is a traditional chinese medical therapy in which moxa (made from dried mugwort *Artemisia argyi*) or other herbs are burnt on, around or above acupuncture pointed. **Moxa** can be rolled into balls, shaped into cones or other forms and then can be burnt directly on the skin or indirectly on a medium (such as ginger, garlic, salt, aconite, pepper, etc.—according to indications) in between the moxa and the skin **(indirect moxibustion)**.

Direct moxibustion method may be blister forming (scarring method) or nonblister forming (nonscarring) method (in which moxa cones are burnt directly on the skin but is removed when burning starts causing intense pain). Burning of moxa is supposed to expel cold and warm the meridians, which thereafter promotes smoother and efficient flow of blood.

Besides various general and specific indications of moxibustion, it has been seen that along with acupuncture or in combination with external cephalic version, moxibustion is effective in changing the breech presentation of babies. In such indication, perhaps the moxibustion causes the release of placental estrogen and prostaglandins, which leads to uterine contractions that helps in changing the position of baby.

The following write up is much based (even copied at places) on the articles of Deepak and Rao 2021. Yoga and meditation as a mind, body and lifestyle interventions has gained popularity in recent times. Ever since the declaration of 21 June as the International Day of Yoga by the United Nations General Assembly in 2014, Yoga, as a health promotion intervention, has gained popularity globally with due support from majority of the nations and the World Health Organization (WHO)—(Deepak and Rao 2021).

The resurgence of COVID-19 in 2021 has enhanced the burden on the healthcare resources in our any country with marked increase in the number of cases. In their cases and even among the healthcare workers, impending anxiety and stress can down regulate immune response and defenses that can lead them to contract this infection and increase in severity. Treatment protocols for people with COVID-19 should address both the physiologically and psychological needs of the patients and health service providers.

There has been evidence that enhancing physical and mental health may reduce burden of acute respiratory illness. Regular physical activity such as moderate exercise may protect people from acute respiratory illness. The recommended means of the aerobic exercise is walking with an optimal frequency of 3–5 days a week and an optimal duration of 20–30 minutes of continuous activity (Glesson et al. 2011). Moderate exercise is known to increase salivary IgA secretion which is known to reduce the risk of infections. Studies on Yoga and meditation in managing the symptoms during Influenzas reason have shown promising results considering that the persons above 50 years are vulnerable to contract infections including COVID illness—Yoga appears to be useful as a preventive measure.

Nearly based on more or less similar theme, Master Choa Kok Sui advocated about PRANIC HEALING which varyingly got popularity. Pranic healing is not intended to replace orthodox medicines, but rather to compliment it by teaching the connection between physical body and the human energy system (aura, chakras and meridians).

Pranic healing is claimed to be a revolutionary healing technique and helps in improving health, happiness, success, and peace. Yoga practices like kriyas, pranayama, and asanas have great role in reducing airways reactivity and enhance respiratory effort in subjects. Yoga and meditative practices can play an important role and adjunct in reducing psychological distress in the community.

CHAPTER 22

Reiki and Yoga

"Focus where it matters."

—SP

"Just as a candle cannot burn without fire,
men (human beings) cannot live without spiritual life."

—Budha

CHAPTER OUTLINE

- Reiki
- Yoga
- Stick as a friend
- Nail to vault yoga (नख शिख योग) (NVY)
- History of materials used for intra-articular injection as in appendix

REIKI

The basic principle of Reiki is based on an idea that an unseen "life energy force" flows through our systems which keep us alive. If this energy force is low, one is more likely to feel sick and depressed, and if it is high, one is more likely to be healthy and happy.

"Reiki" is a Japanese word comprising two components.
'Rei' = Omnipresent + God's wisdom or the higher power
'Ki' = Energy of life - "life force energy"

Rieki is actually spiritually guided life force energy, which is always with us in varied extent.

The **'energy of life'** comes with life and goes with death.

Dr Mikao Usui of Japan reinnovated the process of 'Reiki'—which had been popular in various forms at least in ancient India. The Saint Guru Vasistha (religious teacher and priest of Lord Rama's dynasty) had innovated the process of "Treatment by touch"—*'Sparsh Chikitsa'* which we have forgotten.

The principle of **Reiki** is more or less guided by 'psychosomatic effect'.

They believe that there are seven major energising points *"Chakra"* in the body, of which four located in the upper part of body are triggered to energise the life.

The Reiki system teaches:

- To control the emotions
- To develop self-confidence
- To undermine the symptoms
- To develop the overall psychological power, strength, will and confidence.

Nonorganic diseases, psycho-oriented diseases/symptoms, depressive psychosis, unexplained symptoms, backache, headache and alike conditions have been claimed to have fastly improved under the process of Reiki.

The process of Reiki can be imparted even in two days. It can be self-imparted as well.

Reiki is imparted by laying on hands. During treatment through Reiki one feels a peculiar glowing radiance which flows through one's body and around it. It does not treat just one disease in the body, rather it takes care of the body as a whole including its physique, mind, emotions, spirituality and even the surrounding. After the treatment through Reiki, which is a simple, safe, natural and spiritual healing, one feels relaxed, peaceful, secured, improved, healthy and happy.

Reiki provides guidelines to live a gracious peaceful healthy life.

Reiki is: *"The secret art of inviting happiness.*
The miraculous medicine of all diseases. Just for today, do not anger.
Do not worry and be filled with gratitude.
Devote yourself to your work. Be kind to people.
Every morning and evening, join your hands in prayer.
Pray these words to your heart and chant these words with your mouth. Usui Reiki Treatment for the improvement of body and mind"—The founder, Usui Mikao. The International Centre for Reiki 21421 Hilltop street, unit#28. Southfield, Michigan 48033.

Reiki can be used along with other systems of management and therapies to promote overall recovery.

Reiki is a simple technique to learn, and is transferred to the student during an attunement (accustom/adjust) by a Reiki master. It does not require any super intellectuality to learn it, however, a keen student can acquire the unlimited supply of 'life force energy', which helps in improving one's health, wisdom, spirituality and overall quality of life.

YOGA—THE SOURCE OF QUIETING THE MIND-'ॐ' IS THE GUIDE

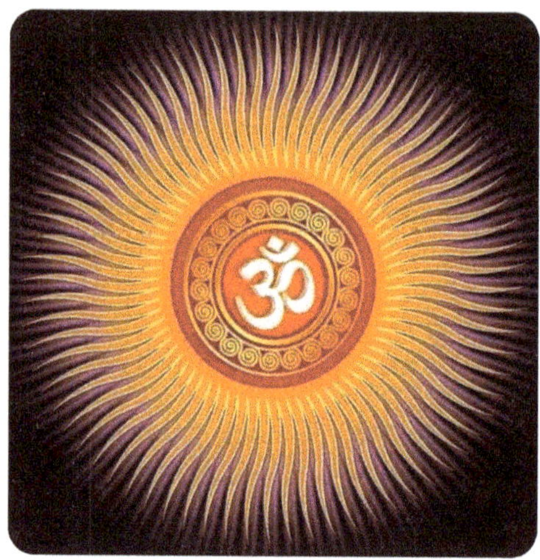

Courtesy: Website___pinterest.com

"*Om*" or "Aum" is the first sound that emerged from the vibrations of the cosmic energy that created the universe. "*Om*" is derived from the ancient Sanskrit language and is believed to be the primordial sound that gave birth to the universe. It is often referred to as "Pranava", which denotes the sound of creation. *Om* is a sacred sound and a spiritual icon and symbol in Hinduism, Buddhism, Jainism, and several religions. It is believed to be the cosmic vibration that permeates everything in the universe, from the smallest atoms to the galaxies.

Om represents the "trinity"—three fundamental aspects of existence—creation, preservation, and dissolution, which are represented by the Hindu trinity of Gods: Brahma (the creator), Vishnu (the preserver), and Shiva (the destroyer). The three sounds within "*Om*"—A, U, and M—represent the above told aspects, respectively. It is taken as a sacred symbol.

For a lay person, it is synonymous to the meditation and as a doorway to tranquility for yogic practitioners. Chanting or meditating on the sound of "*Om*" brings about a sense of peace, harmony, and connection with the divine. In the process of chanting or meditating, the muscles of body automatically start being toned up, to assume the posture for concentration.

The vibrations created by chanting "*Om*" are thought to have a harmonizing effect on the physical, mental, and spiritual aspects of the person. Regular chanting of "*Om*" morning-evening for a fixed period improves concentration of mind, posture of physique, built of body and self-realization; reduces the stress; and enhances the overall well-being.

The present studies show that even a brief chanting of "*Om*" (about 5 minutes) might enhance the parasympathetic nervous system actively, promote relaxation, and provide calmness. (PubMed central).

"Strength does not come with physical capacity. It comes from indomitable will."
—**Mahatma Gandhi**

"Yoga and meditation help in improving compassion, harmony and all-around progress for the human race besides building and developing one own body, mind and conscience."
— **Narendra Modi**

According to the Chamber's 20th century dictionary 'Yoga' means a system of Hindu philosophy showing the means of emancipation of the soul from further migrations.

Yoga philosophy is one of the six major orthodox schools of Hinduism. It is closely related to the Samkhya School of Hinduism. It teaches control of the mind, senses and body in order to achieve union with God. Yoga systematically shows the ways to enhance oneself physically, mentally, environmentally and spiritually. It helps us to know our inner self, strengthens our inner power and prepares us to attain the eternal bliss.

Yoga is neither a religion, nor a belief, nor a community, but a planned method of leading one's life to achieve a healthy body, peaceful mind and useful life. Yoga is a practical science of self-realization and its regular honest practice (*abhyas*) is the very essence of this science. Fortunately, on the suggestion of Hon'ble Shri Narendra Modi, the Prime Minister of India, the United Nations has declared 21st of June as "The International Yoga Day". The Yoga is now being practiced in about 170 countries or even more.

The origin of yoga is very deep rooted and is found in the most sacred ancient religious literature of Hindus—The Vedas. The Rig Veda (Hymn 5.81.1) defines the 'Yoga' as a dedication to the rising sun in the morning (*Savitri*) interpreted as 'Yoke' or 'yogically controlled.' The '*Yoga Sutras*' of sage '*Patanjali*' written approximately in AD 200 as a '*Yoga Darshan*' is a key text of the Yoga School of Hinduism.

The 'Bhagavad Gita'—the most universally accepted religious sacred text of India written in 3rd or 4th century BC—contains 700 verses depicting the practical philosophy of yoga-based or '*Karma Yog*', i.e., universal concept of **'you reap what you sow'** as the basic law of '*Karma*'.

Sage Patanjali describes the fundamental ethical perceptions as '*Yamas*' and '*Niyamas* (rules)', which guide us about the ways of observing the universal morality to optimally shape our attitude and develop our proper relationship to others and ourselves.

Yamas guide us about the 'dos and don'ts' in our universal dealings, moral disciplines and restraints and regulary remind us about our fundamental nature, which is honest, generous, compassionate and peace-loving. *Yamas* also regularly show us the path of honesty, peaceful living, nonviolence (*Ahimsa*), commitment to truthfulness (*Satya*), non-stealing habit (*asteya*), respectful and truthful honor of other's trust in us, moderation and self-control in sex and the senses (*Brahmacharya*), and not being greedy nor to have tendency of hoarding.

'*Niyamas*' (the rules of laws) regulate and discipline our life with self restraints creating a code for living healthy, soulfully, peacefully with modesty, satisfaction and spirituality. Devotion to one's work, sincere efforts, the spiritual path and the feet of the Almighty is quite essential to achieve the ultimate goal.

The regular practice of the path of yoga ultimately leads to a truthful, healthy and useful life. Broadly, the common major paths of yoga are:

1. *Karma Yoga*—the path of selfless service which is the essence of teachings of Gita.
2. *Bhakti Yoga*—the path of devotion and total surrender to the feet of God.
3. *Raj Yoga*—the path of controlling the mind which is popularly known as 'Yoga.'

It is also known as '*Ashtanga Yoga*' or the yoga of eight steps/practices. Saint Patanjali depicts eight yogic practices (*Ashtang Yog*) as follows:

"यमनियमासनप्राणायामप्रत्याहारधायणाध्यानसमाध्यअष्टौअडर्गानि"

—Yog Darshan 2/29

That is—*Yam* (resistance to passions); *Niyam* (rules); *Asana* (postures); *Pranayam* (controlled exercise of breathing); *Pratyahar* (resistance to senses); *Dharana* (concentration); *Dhyan* (meditation); *Samadhi* (union with the infinite) are the eight principles of Yoga.

Asana (Postures) (Figures 22.1 to 22.19)

Sitting in a particular assigned posture (after being tested for longer period is called '*asana*', such as *Padmasan, Bhadrasan, Sarpasan, Sidhasan, Sukhasan*, etc. *Hathyoga* describes 84 types of *asans*. The *asans* must be practiced regularly, calmly, comfortably, devotionally for optimum period sitting on a thinly cushioned mat (such as a piece of blanket) in the fresh air environment of morning. Meditations and worships performed in well-practiced *asans* increase the concentration and peace of mind and also makes the body agile, flexible, active and healthy.

Meditation is a process of relaxing in God's will. During this process and duration, one should (and can) forget all our wants, ambitions and desires. Meditation (*dhyaan*) is a way of religiously focusing one's mind upon an activity to achieve a mental status free from emotional turbulence and mental distraction. One should just sit in a receptive mood and accept what God thinks is best for us. Ultimately, one will find that God gives much more than what was desired and expected.

Examples of few commonly practiced Asanas are given below (**Figures 22.1 to 22.7**) based on the courtesy of Swami Ramdev ji.

"Kriya Yoga is the solution in these times of pollution."

Kriya yoga emphasises deep and measured breathing. Kriya yoga is a holistic system and may be incorporated in our lifestyle harmonising with our all other activities. In a period of continuous practice our body becomes a system of automatic filtering activity constantly neutralizing negative currents and producing positive prana. This auto-cleaninsing continues even when we enter into any toxic environment.

Note: The above written broad outline of the yoga philosophy is based on the publications of:

1. *"The divine life society"* PO Shivanandanagar, 249,192, Uttarakhand, Himalayas, India.
2. *"Yog Its Philosophy and Practice"* by Swami Ramdev, Divya, Prakashan, Kankhal, Haridwar, Uttarakhand, 249,408.
3. Photographs of '*asans*' are based on the illustrations given in the book—*Yog its Philosophy and Practice* by Swami Ramdev ji. (By permission)
4. Inner voice of the Hindustan Times.

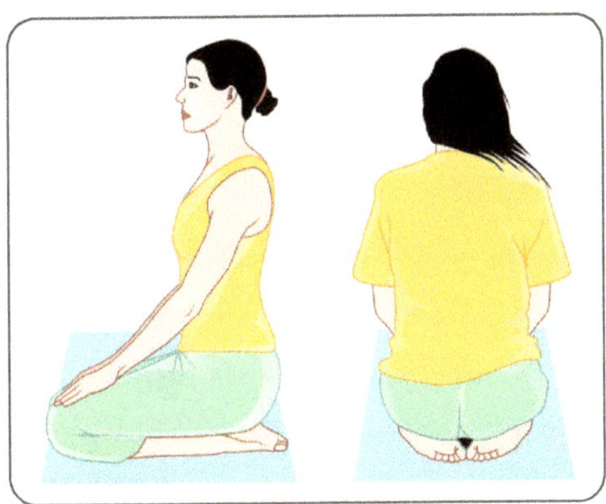

FIG. 22.1: *Vajrasan*: This asan can be done even after meals. It is done to meditate and improve the concentration of mind.

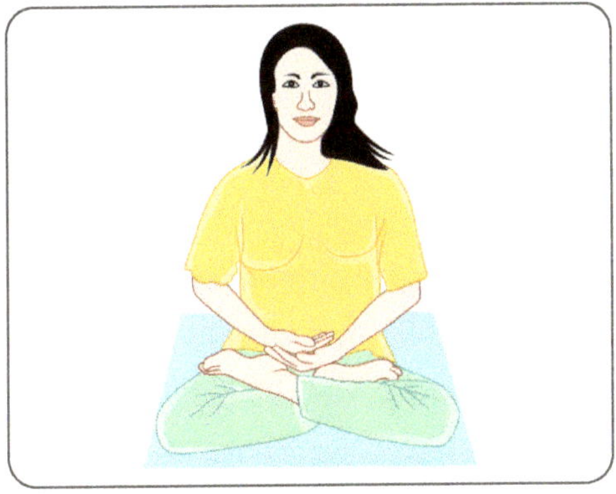

FIG. 22.2: *Padmasan*: It is the best posture for doing meditation. It enhances the concentration of mind. It is useful in dyspepsia and anorexia.

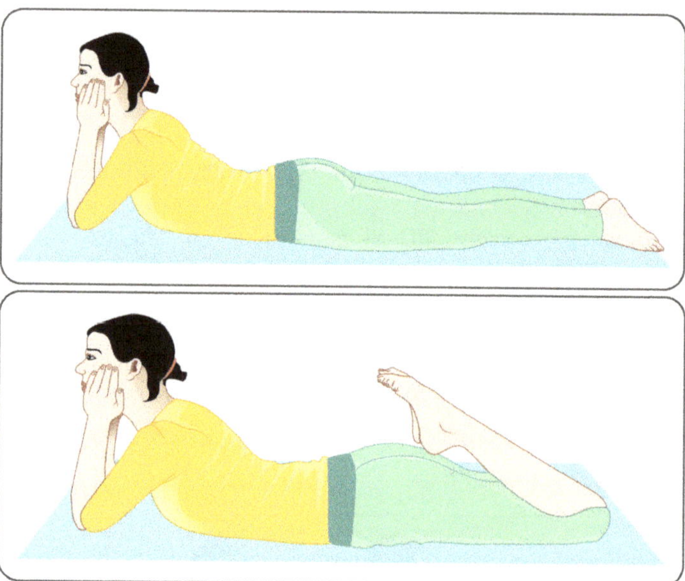

FIG. 22.3: *Makarasan*: It is useful in managing chronic lung diseases like 'asthma'. It is also helpful in chronic spinal problems like intervertebral disc prolapse, degenerative changes in spine.

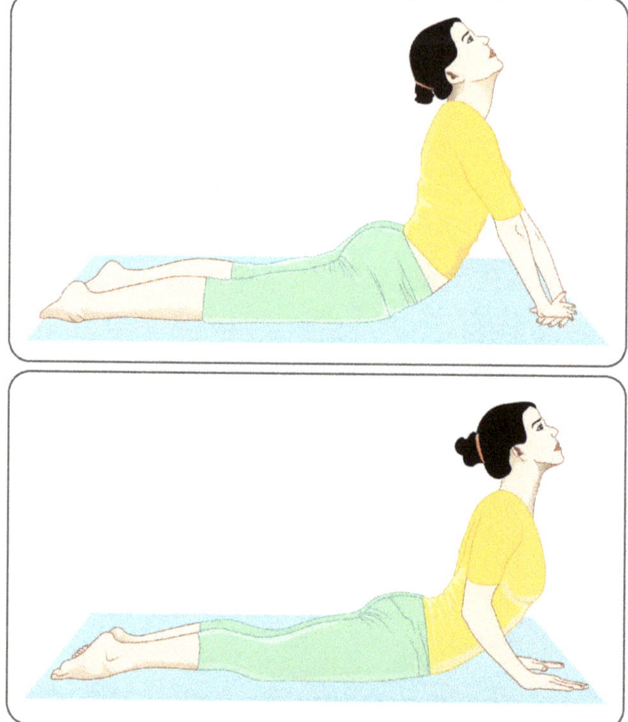

FIG. 22.4: *Bhujangasan*: It is helpful in managing the chronic spinal problems especially related to cervical (like cervical spondylosis) and lumbar regions (such as lumbar spondylosis, chronic disc pathology, ankylosing spondylitis).

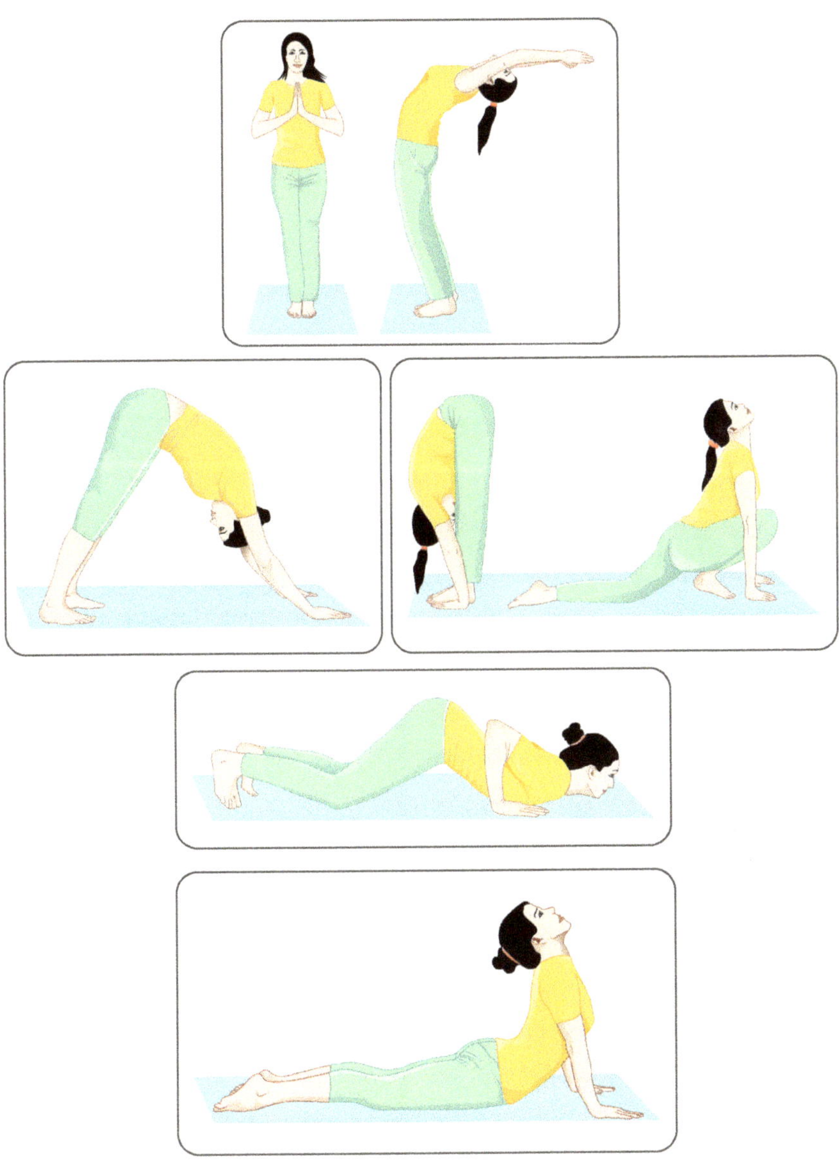

FIG. 22.5: *Surya Namaskar*: These are the wholesome exercises for almost all parts of body including the vital organs and gastrointestinal system. These exercises make the body flexible, strong, energetic and overall healthy.

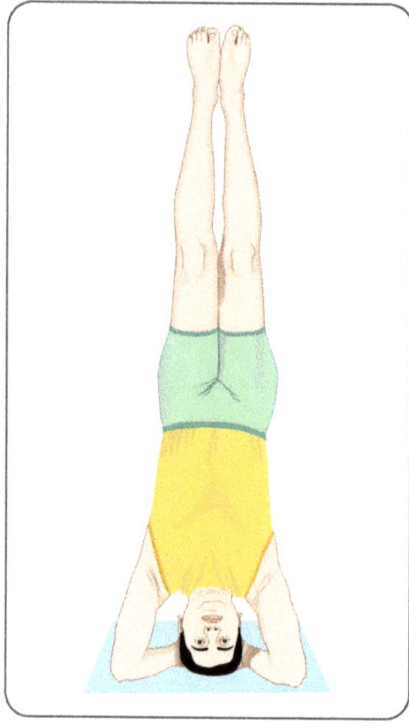

FIG. 22.6: *Shirshasan*: It increases the blood circulation of brain and facial region. It is supposed to enhance the memory, concentration of mind, intelligence and sharpness of mind. However, it should not be done by elderly person, and also the persons with coronary, eye, ear, blood pressure, thyroid and neck problems. Persons who want to do this asan should be otherwise ailment-free.

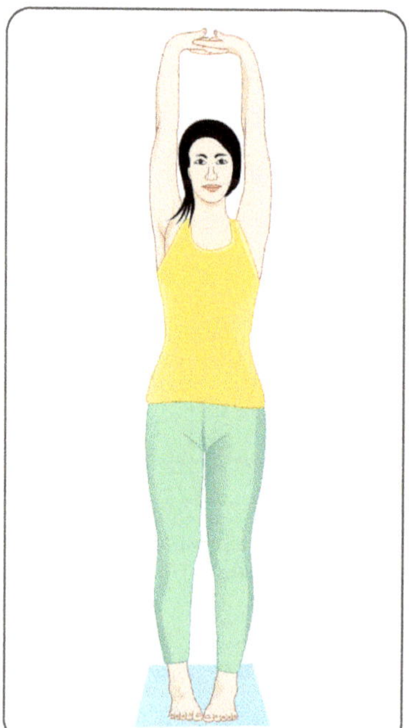

FIG. 22.7: *Tadasan*: In this asan, the person, standing on her fore-feet, stretches her almost the whole body (lower limbs, abdomen, chest, neck and upper limbs) while taking deep breath, and after staying in this posture for sometime (according to her capacity) comes down keeping the feet flat on the ground. The posture is repeated for ten times.

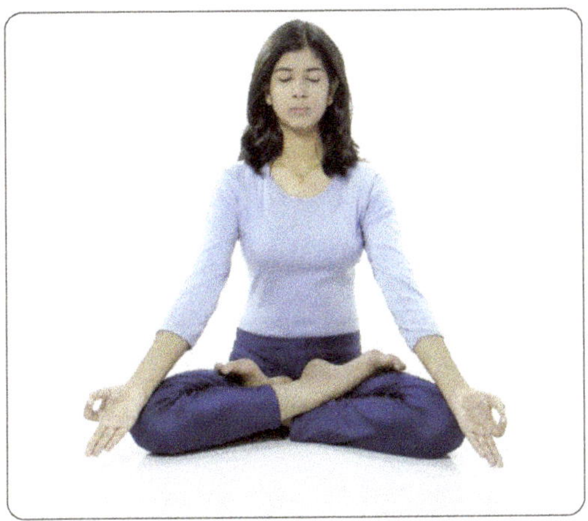

FIG. 22.8: *Bhastrika Pranayama*

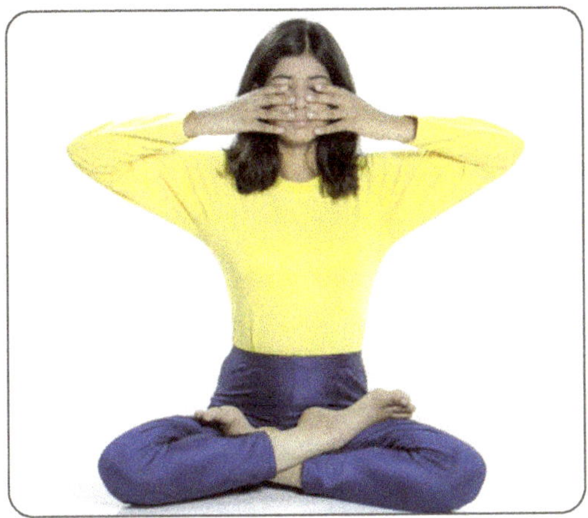

FIG. 22.9: *Bhramari Pranayama*

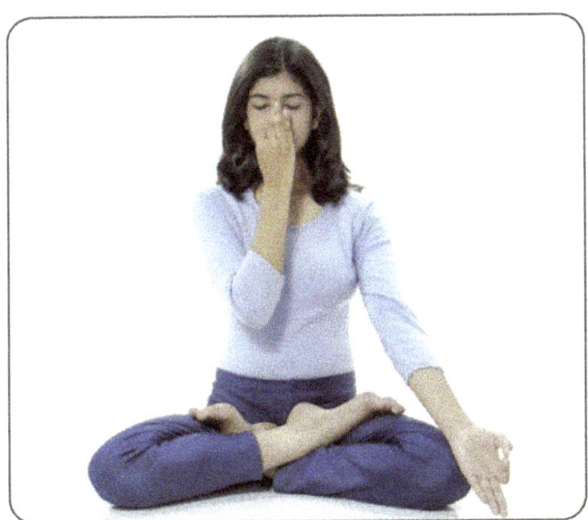

FIG. 22.10: *Nadi Shodhan Pranayama*

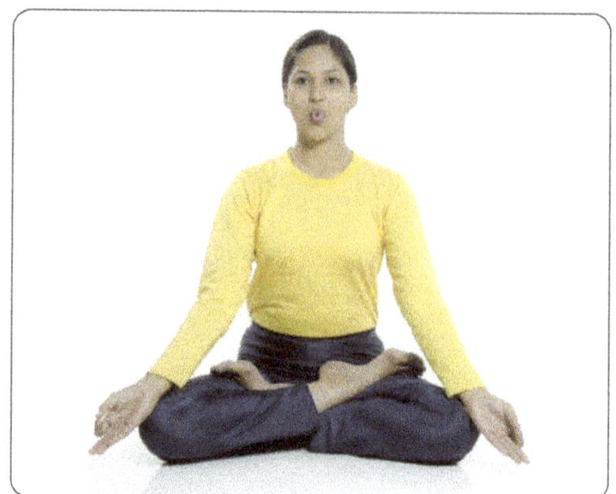

FIG. 22.11: *Shitali Pranayama*

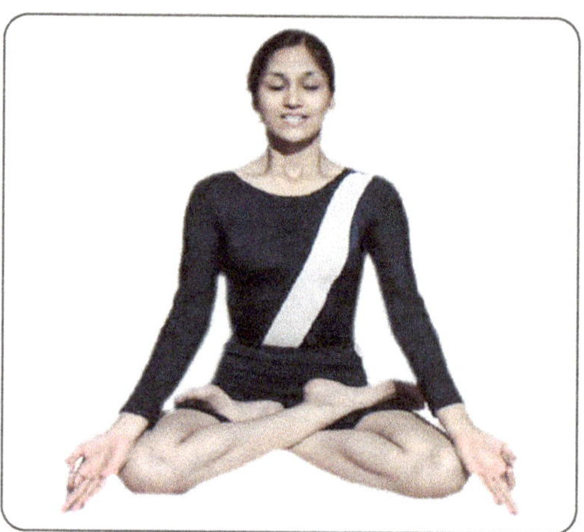

FIG. 22.12: *Sheetkari Pranayama*

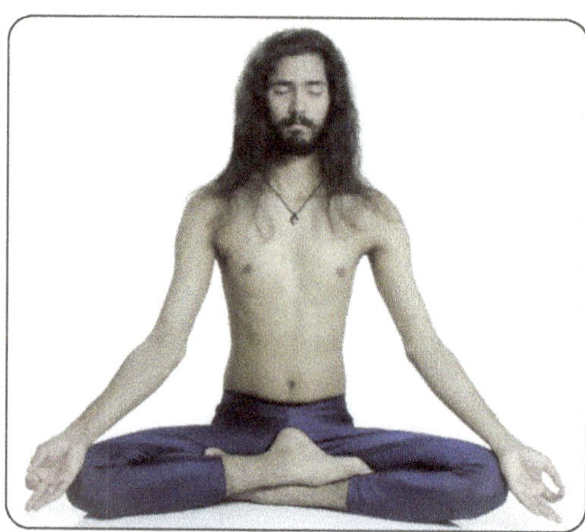

FIG. 22.13: *Siddhasana*

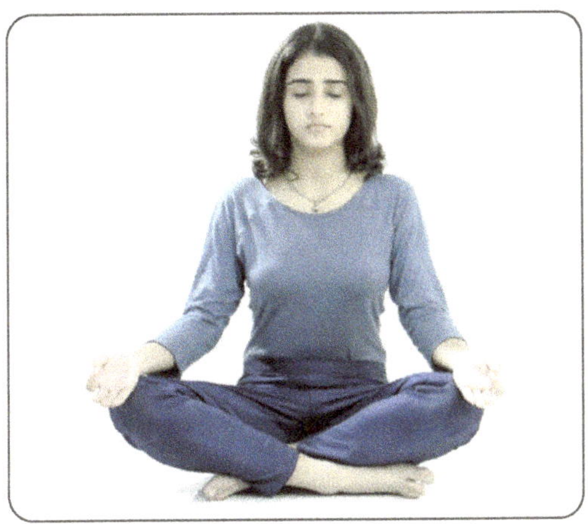

FIG. 22.14: *Sukhasana*

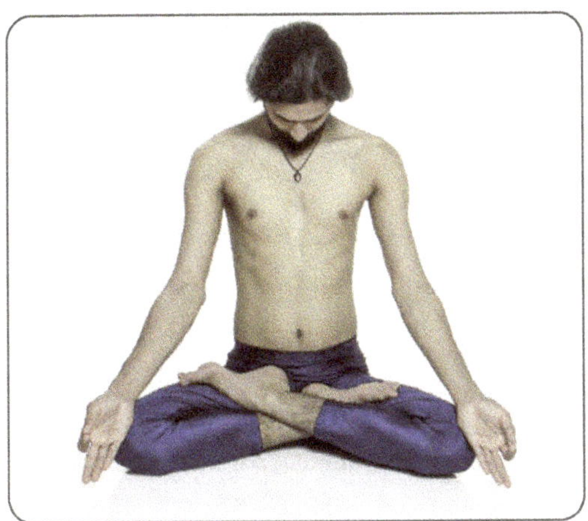

FIG. 22.15: *Ujjayi pranayama*

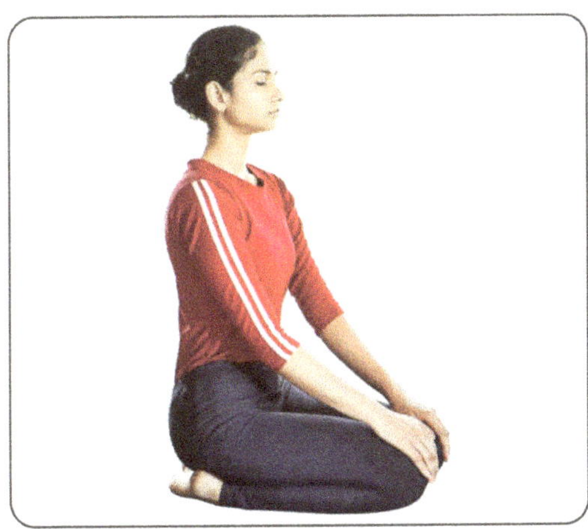

FIG. 22.16: *Vajrasana*

PRANAYAMA

Indians are practicing प्राणायाम (Pranayama) since thousands of years. Its knowledge was transmitted through mouth, say from the great ancient "Yoga Gurus" (teachers). Those teachers have practiced the system and realized their utility. They concluded that "Pranayama" is one of the most useful and important practices of "*Hathyog*" Patanjali Yog Sutra. The practices of "pranayama" should be started after attaining perfection in "*Padmasan*". Pranayama is the eighth wing of "Patanjali Yog Sutra" or fourth wing of "*Ashtang Yog*".

Pranayama forms a useful part of yogic practices. It is a science of yogic practice which remains useful in regularizing the respiratory system throughout life. The main aim of Pranayama is to regularize the respiratory system in a controlled way and thereafter affects the concentration of the central nervous system and works of mind.

Pranayama involves three phases (processes)—rapid respiration (पूरक), stopping of respiration (कुम्भक), and almost complete release of respiration (रेचक). The above three respiratory activities regularize the flow of energy and life in every useful part of body.

Pranayama should be practiced in open, airy, and healthy environment. For a beginner, Pranayama should be started in March-April or September-October, and thence should be continued as yoga practice regularly.

Yoga pranayama should be done in the morning after sitting on a comfortable mildly cushioned seat (आसन).

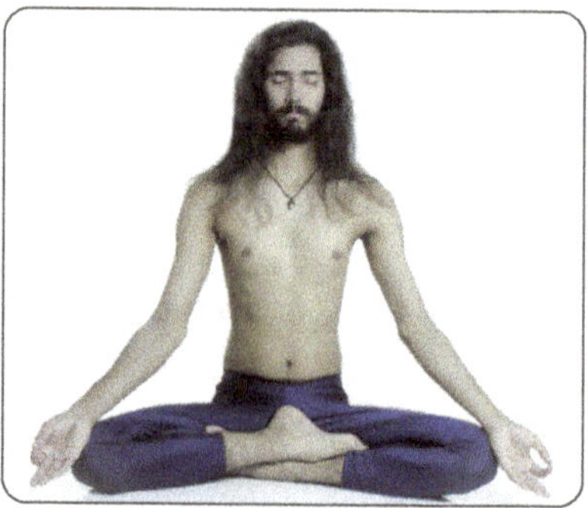

Fig. 22.17: *Siddhasana*

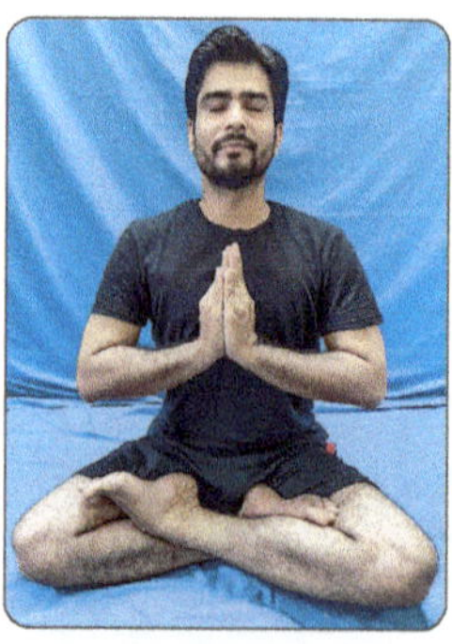

FIG. 22.18: *Padmasana*

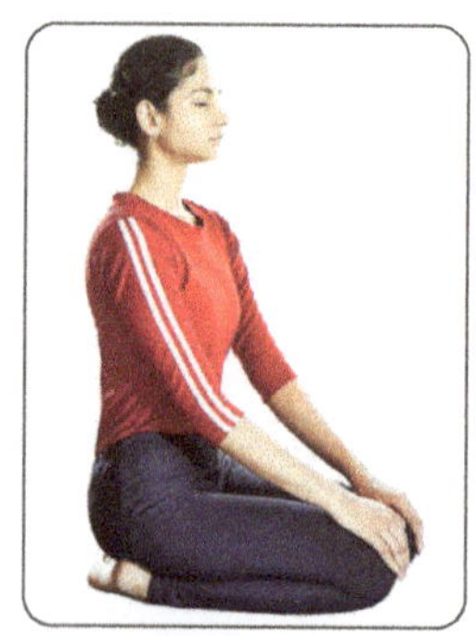

Fig. 22.19: *Vajrasana*

STICK AS A FRIEND

1. Sticks as confident friend for elder people: When one retires from active service/job/profession (about 65 years of age), one should use walking stick (with one leg) as his/her company—as confident friend **(Figure 22.20)**.

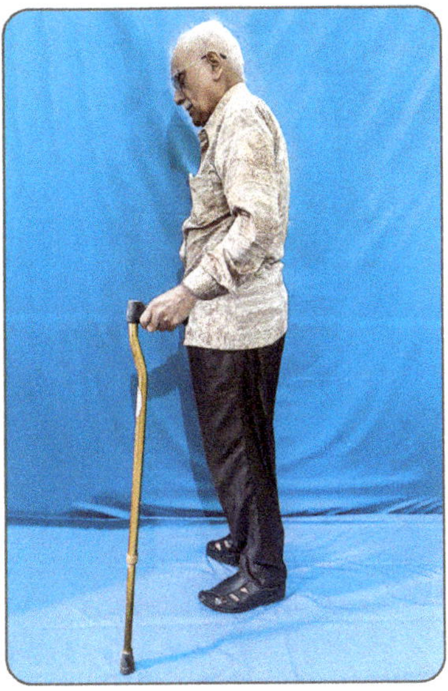

FIG. 22.20: Stick 1

2. When one further retires from his/her active household activities, one should use stick with tri/quadripod **(Figure 22.21)**. Use of two sticks **(Figure 22.22)** increases the stability (mainly in the rotatory instability) on even or uneven ground.

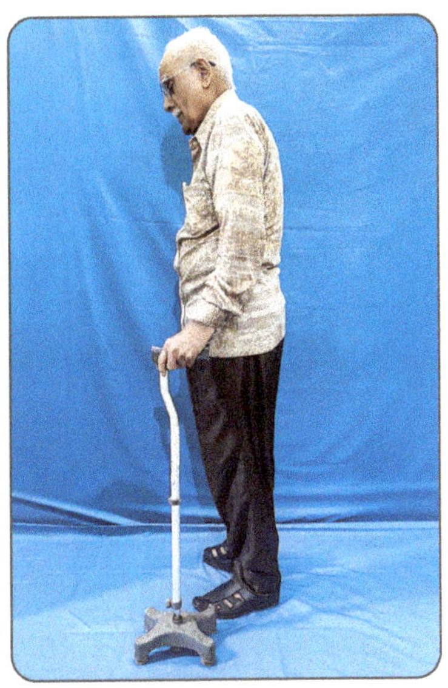

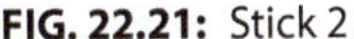

FIG. 22.21: Stick 2

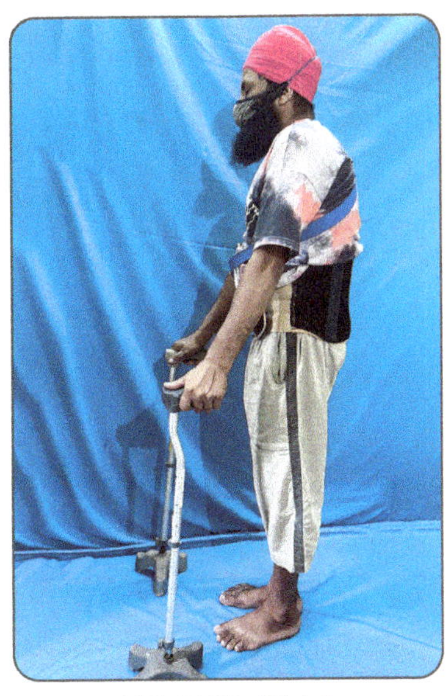

FIG. 22.22: Stick 3

3. It is always better to use walker [with four stable legs and with anti-slippery rubber ferrule while going to washroom/bathroom **(Figure 22.23)**].

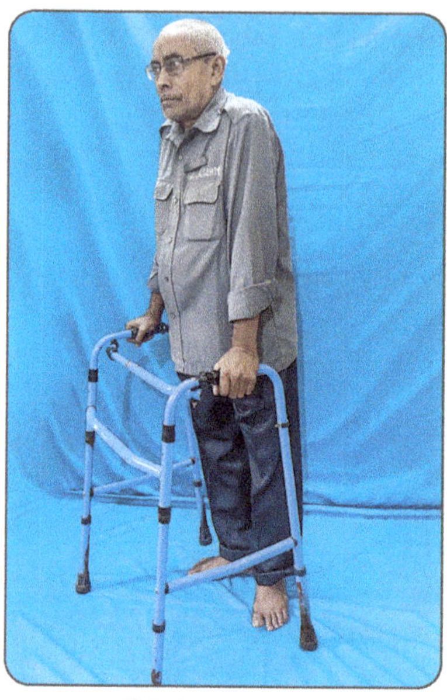

FIG. 22.23: Stick 4

For improving the stability of a body perform the following exercises: Hold the head board of the bed or the back support of the chair firmly **(Figure 22.24)**.

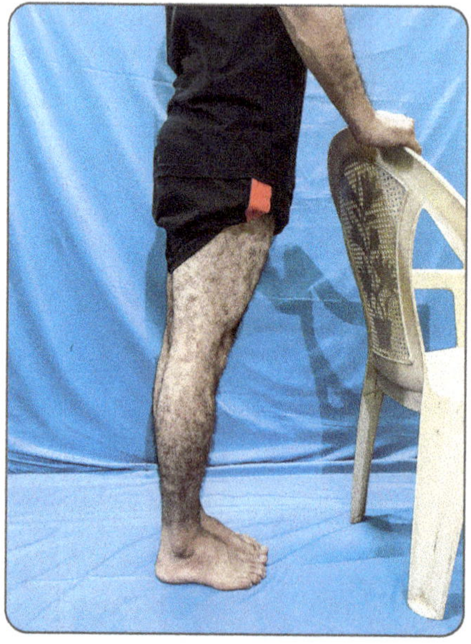

FIG. 22.24: Stability 1

Stand vertically straight first on both legs and lift your heels fully **(Figure 22.25)**, and sustain in the position for 15–20 seconds and then, fold one bent knee firmly and fully **(Figure 22.26)**, stay in this position for 10 seconds, then change this activity to other leg alternately (20–30 times).

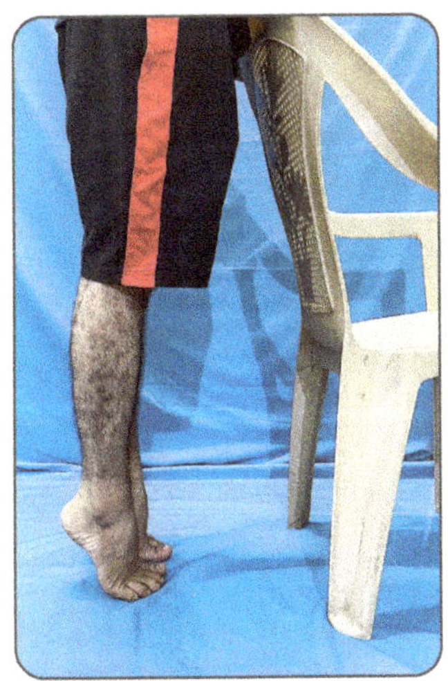

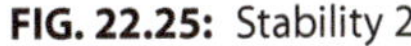

FIG. 22.25: Stability 2

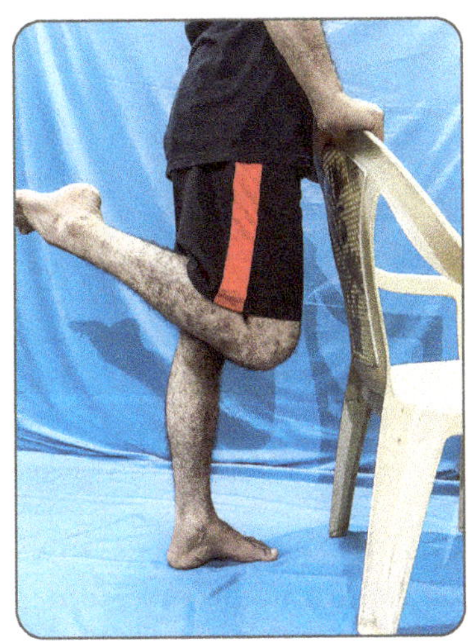

FIG. 22.26: Stability 3

NAIL TO VAULT YOGA (NVY) नख शिख योग (नशयो) (FIGURES 22.27 TO 22.69)

Now Yoga has become/is becoming the essential part of living schedules to keep one fairly physically fit in the life. Various types and programs of Yoga processes/practices have been scheduled and practiced.

With advancing age, one should avoid sitting on the floor, squatting as far as possible and also the Buddha-position sitting, unless one has practiced these through his/her young age.

Sitting in **90-90-90** position **(Figure 22.27)** in the advance age most likely helps in maintaining the posture of back and lower limbs, tones the muscles of back and lower limbs, in performing most of the needed exercises of the lower limbs. It helps in improving the concentration of mind, e.g., meditation.

As the age advances toward the older age one should accordingly reduce the vigorous activities/exercises/running/yoga and strenuous practices like "*Shirshasan*". However, the moderate and practical yoga schedules should be practiced regularly and on the whole, it proves to be practical, helpful and non-exertive. The "NVY" practices have been recommended to be practiced mainly by the **elderly persons** who should avoid going for any gym-activity, unaided (without stick) walking especially on unsafe crowded roads or even irregular surfaces of garden. Sitting cross-legged [in Buddha position/ *Padmasan* **(Figure 22.28)**] is good, but unless practiced from beginning this regularly, it is a strained sitting.

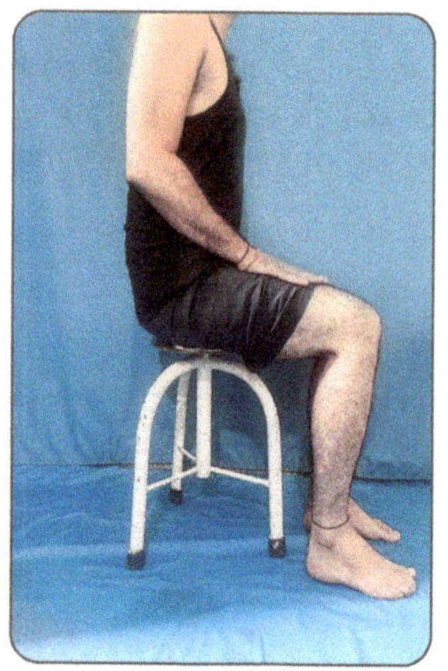

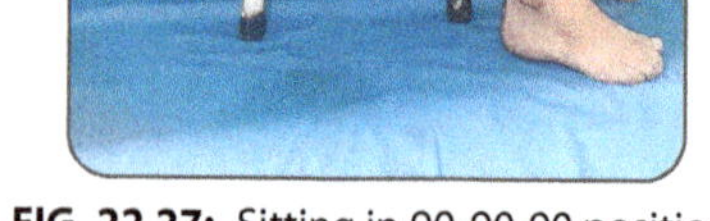

FIG. 22.27: Sitting in 90-90-90 position.

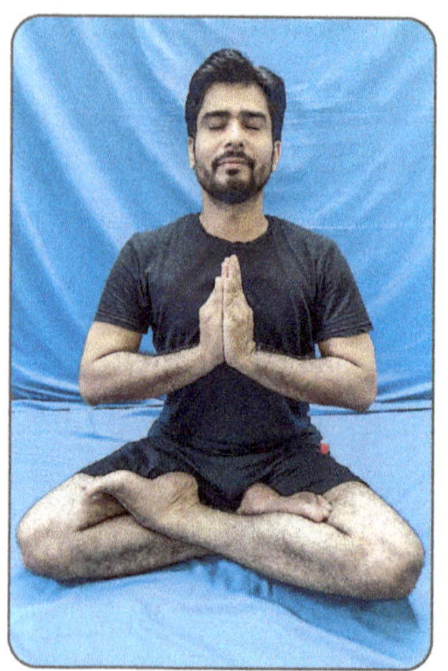

FIG. 22.28: NVY

The principles involved in the NVY processes have been:

A. Initially practice to sit on firm cot/couch/chairs with arms, with hip bent at 90°, knees bent at 90° and feet planted on the floor, which prevents undergoing any risk of road hazards or risks of falling. In this position start with swinging the 90° bent knees in and out for about a minute (i.e., adducting and abducting at hips). The actions noted above make you sit properly, preparing yourself for performing Yoga activities. **(Figures 22.29 to 22.31)**

B. Almost all physical activities of parts of body [feet, ankles, knees, hips, pelvis, spine, abdomen, chest, cardiovascular system; indirectly upper limbs (shoulders, elbows, forearms, hands including fingers and

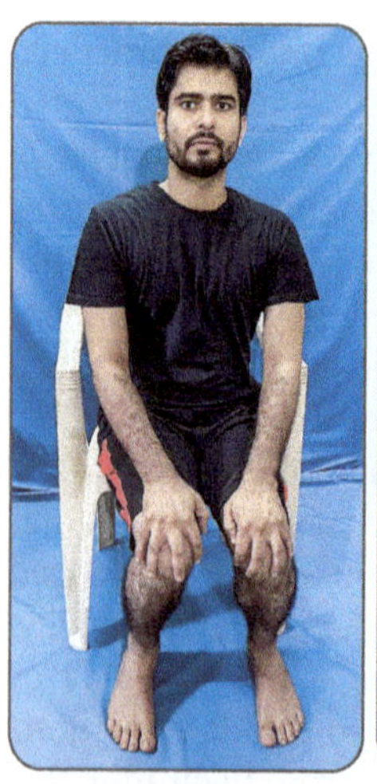

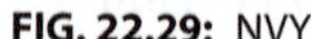

FIG. 22.29: NVY

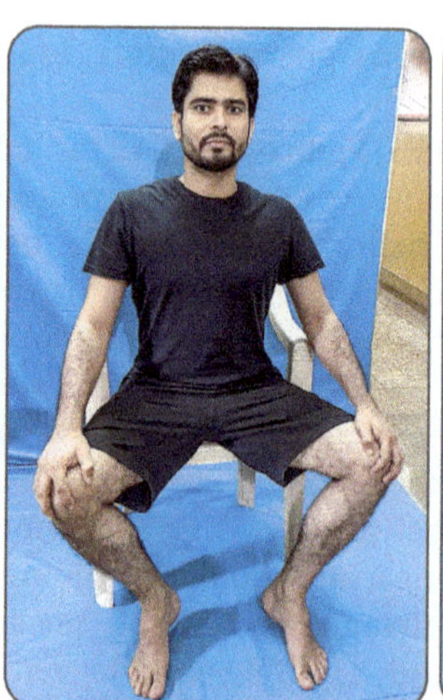

FIG. 22.30: NVY

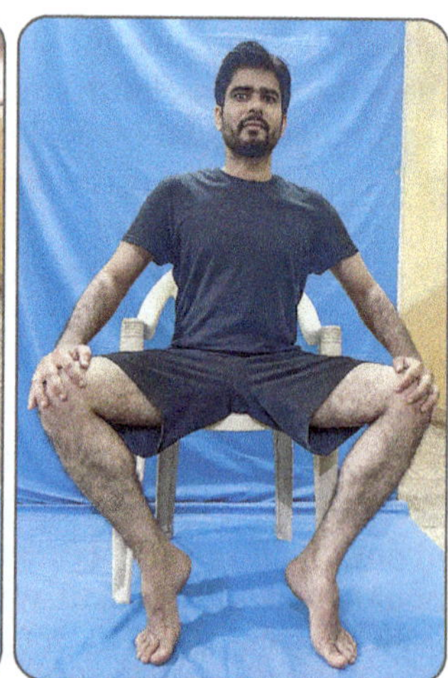

FIG. 22.31: NVY

thumbs)] are taken careof during the yoga exercises and which at the same time bring them to use as needed, since in this '*Nakh Shikh Yoga*' (Nail to Vault Yoga) activities almost all organs of the body, are supposed to be actively involved to varying extent.

C. It has been named as 'Nail to Vault Yoga' (नख–शिख योग): Since as mentioned above almost all physical parts of body are made to be involved—to mild-to-moderate use/activity—in performing the yogas.

D. This should be practiced daily regularly—preferably in the morning (at least 5 days a week for about 45-50 minutes), that covers all the regions to well acceptable level. It is helpful to do each exercise in numerically counted numbers like 20/50/100/150/200 times and keep the routine continued in same fashion. In the beginning, if it is difficult to achieve the desired numbers, begin with smaller numbers like 10, 15, 20....... and gradually increase it according to capacity and endurance.

The process should be started from the distal part of feet and proceed proximally almost joint-wise like ankles, calf (calves), knees, hips (including pelvis), spine (back-abdomen-chest)—and they involve almost simultaneously, upper limbs (shoulders, elbows, forearms, wrists, hands, fingers, thumbs).

Proceed as follows for NVY:

1. The process is started from the distal most portions of feet, i.e., toes - in the first step—the intrinsic muscles of the feet and dorsiflexors and plantar flexors of feet are commissioned to work—

   Do flexion and inversion of both whole feet as one unit as far as possible ⇄ and then eversion and dorsiflexion of whole feet as far as possible. **(Figures 22.32 and 22.33)**.

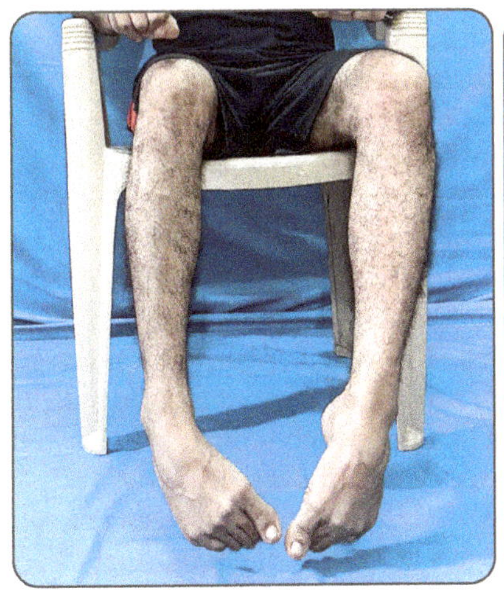

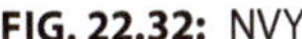
FIG. 22.32: NVY

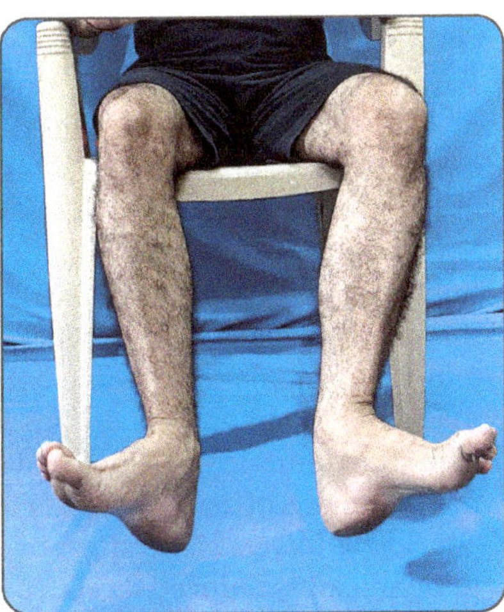

FIG. 22.33: NVY

2. Maximum dorsiflexion and plantar flexion of ankles →
   a. Without touching the heels on the ground
   b. The same as above while the heels touch on ground.

   The muscles involved in dorsiflexon and plantar flexion of the ankles are put to action and ankle joint functions to full extent **(Figures 22.34 and 22.35)**.

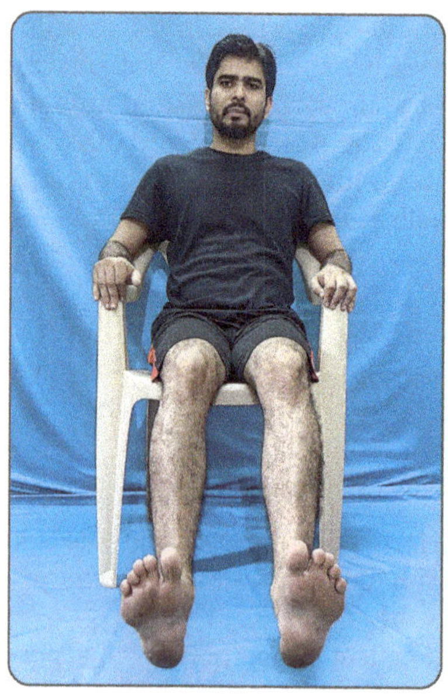

FIG. 22.34: NVY

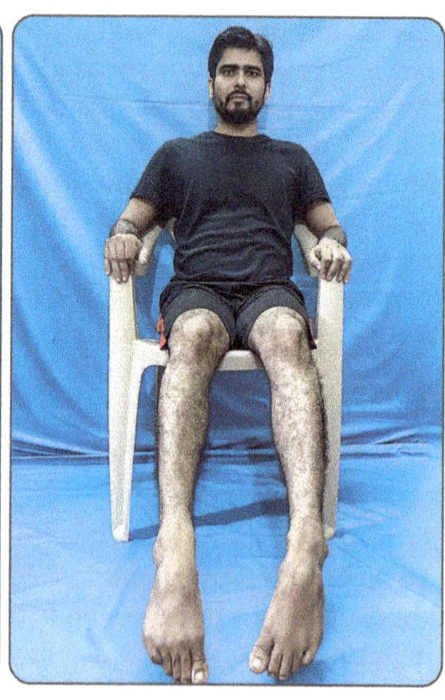

FIG. 22.35: NVY

3. **Soleus push-up:** Sit at the edge of the couch or on a firm wooden chair with trunk firmly erect and soles of feet just resting on the floor, and knees bent at 90°. Lift the heels up to the maximum, while the front parts of soles press on the floor. Sustain in this position for 5-10 seconds—go back to the position of whole soles resting on the floor. Repeat the process at regular intervals. In 90° bent knee, gastrocnemius is made off, and Soleus only functions to plantar flex the ankle. In this action Soleus is very important to pump the venous blood upwards toward the heart. Thus, this exercise helps in improving the functions of cardiovascular system and partly pulmonary system as well. This Soleus push-up if done after meals the blood propels toward the muscles and increase the activities of muscles, thus lessens the need of insulin, which indirectly helps in the managements of diabetics too **(Figures 22.36 and 22.37)**.

   The Soleus lowers blood sugar by its' inability to store glycogen or keep it to significantly reduced levels, so it gets its source of energy/fuel directly from the bloodstream, the glucose, lowering it as it consumes the excess blood sugar—(Daniel Ofodile).

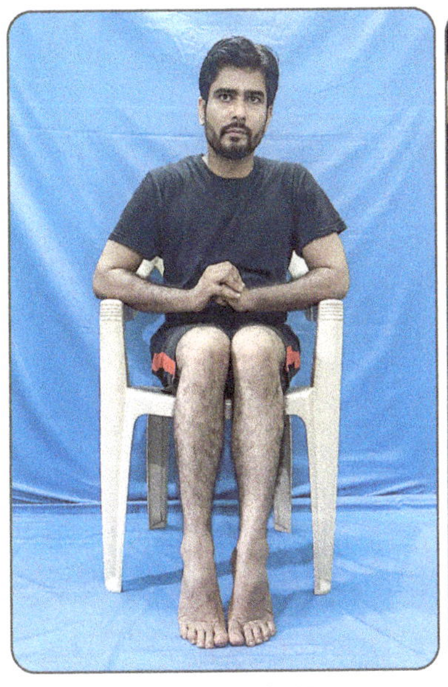

FIG. 22.36: NVY

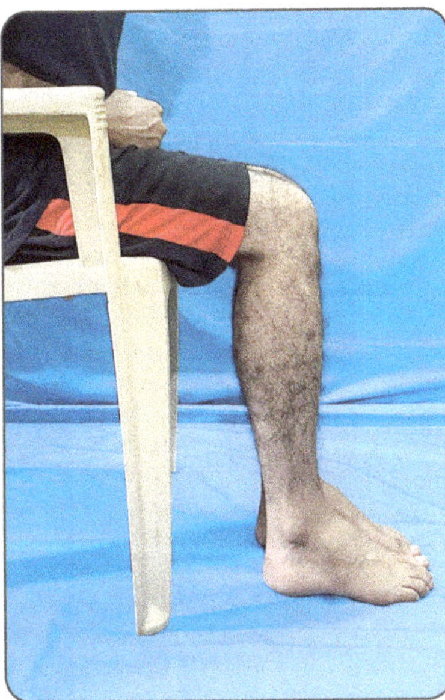

FIG. 22.37: NVY

4. Sit at the edge of couch or on a firm wooden chair with back of lower thighs resting on the edge of couch—flex the knees by about 60° and then extend the knees to zero position. Repeat the positions of knees like pendulum (from flexion to extension).

   The **flexion and extension of knees**, if repeatedly done definitely develop the quadriceps and knee flexor muscles, thus it increases the knee functions, the knee range of motion and the stability of knees.
5. Lying flat on the couch in supine position, extend the hips as much as possible with elevating the buttocks from the couch, and taking purchase at the back of both flexed elbows and both heels **(Figures 22.38 to 22.40)**. This maneuver stretches and develops the extensors of buttocks, hips and lower spine.

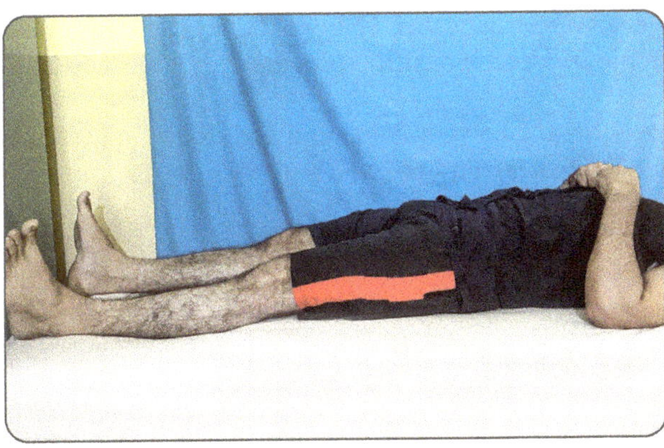

FIG. 22.38: NVY

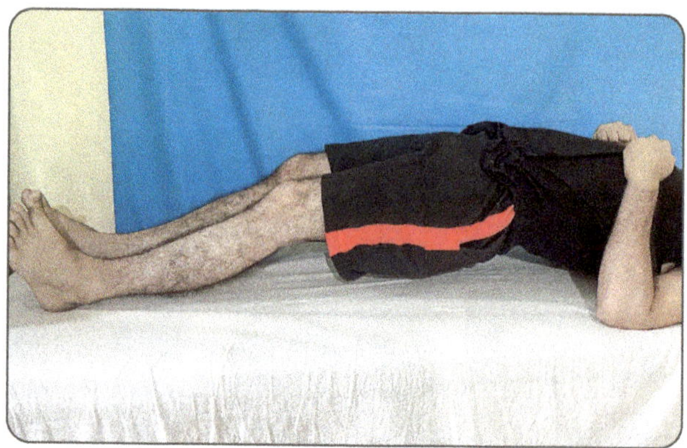

FIG. 22.39: NVY

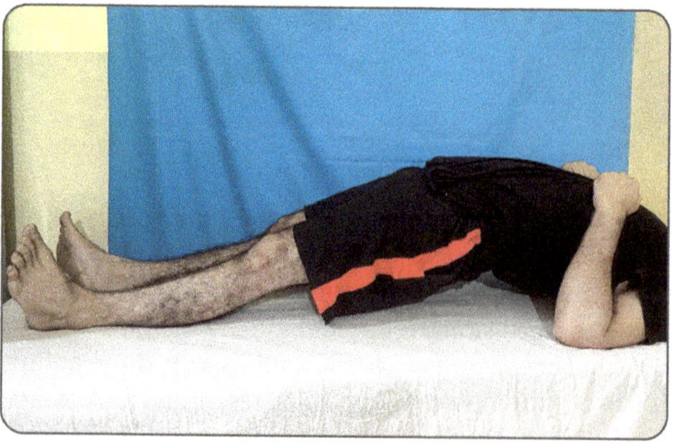

FIG. 22.40: NVY

6. Sit erect at the edge of couch or on a firm wooden chair—extend both lower limbs (with extended knees to zero position, and ankles at zero or fully plantar flexed), abduct the extended lower limbs at the hips - to full extent **(Figure 22.41)**- and then adduct lower limbs fully crossing each other like scissor blades **(Figure 22.42)** then go back to abducted positions of hips, and repeat the process to 30–100 times or as much as you can.

   The power and range of abduction and adduction and stability of hips get improved. The gait is also stabilized and its pattern is improved with these activities.

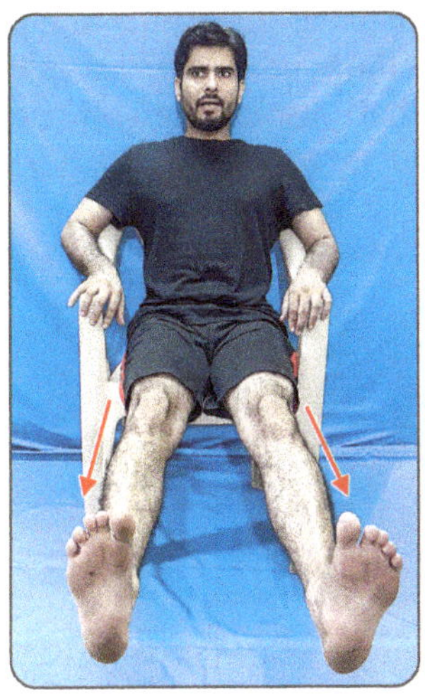

FIG. 22.41: NVY

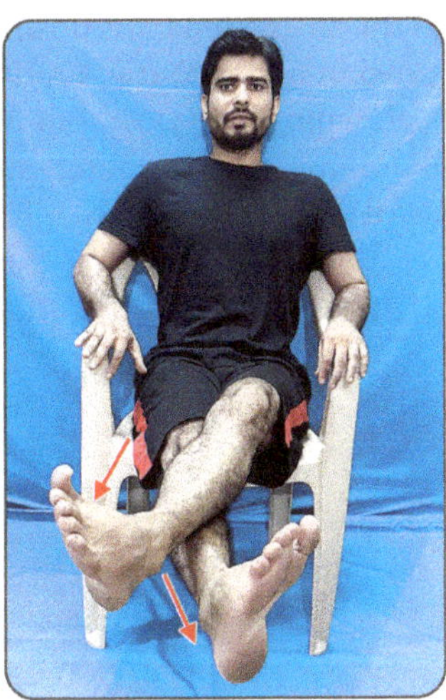

FIG. 22.42: NVY

7. a. Sit erect at the edge of couch or on a stool—take both extended upper limbs at shoulder to the back of pelvis. In this position one hand holds the other wrist and fisted hand, tighten the back, maintain in this position for 10 seconds and then release the tension, and repeat the process for 20-50 times or more which you can do regularly **(Figures 22.43 and 22.44)**.
   b. In the same position as above in the **Figures 22.43 and 22.44** take the held wrists and hands upward up to the lower chest region. In this position diaphragm and abdominal muscles contract and take the

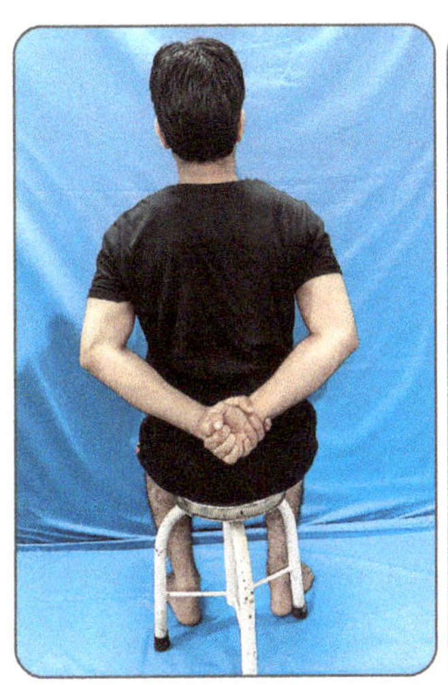

FIG. 22.43: NVY

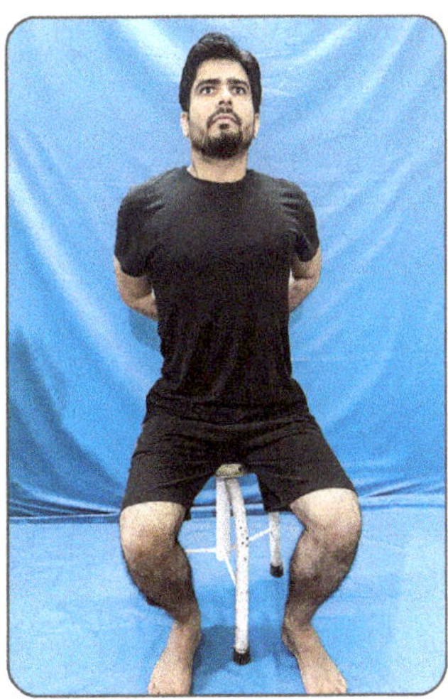

FIG. 22.44: NVY

lungs upwards—hold this position for 10–20 seconds and then release the tension and repeat it 50–100 times or as you can. In this form of yoga, the spinal muscles, abdominal muscles, chest muscles, activities of abdominal viscera, lungs and to varying extent heart activities improve **(Figure 22.45)**.

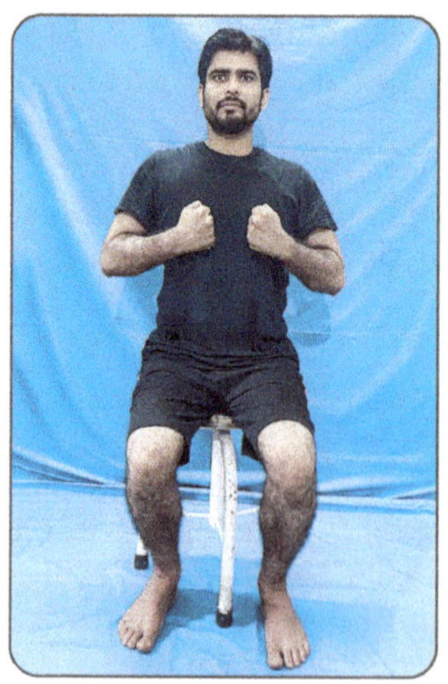

FIG. 22.45: NVY

The strength and stability of upper limbs as a whole and the adduction and flexion of shoulders also get improved.

The hands are fisted, elbows are bent 90°, shoulders are flexed. In these postures the upper limbs are crossed to each other to maximum extent in front of chest repeatedly for about 50–100 times **(Figures 22.46 and 22.47)**.

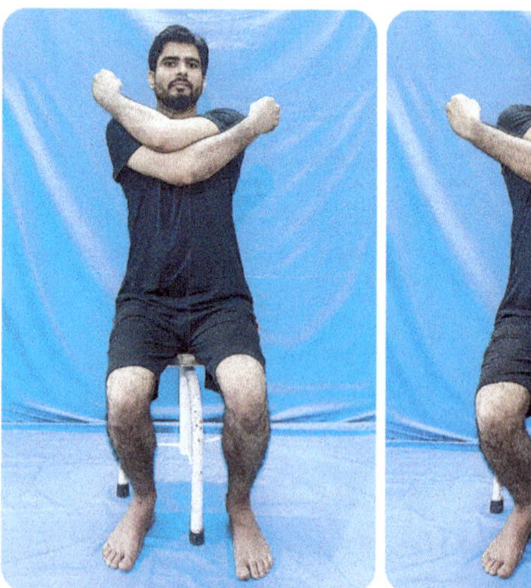

FIG. 22.46: NVY

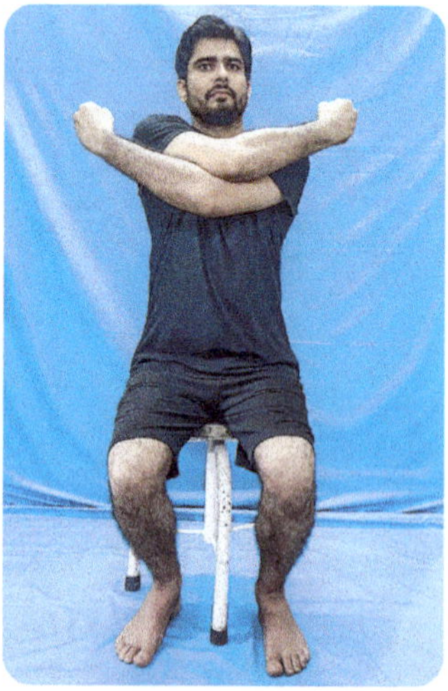

FIG. 22.47: NVY

When both upper limbs with palms and fingers locked in, and taken above the head and brought down to in between the upper part of thighs, the range of motion of shoulders and the strength of controlling muscles improve almost full range of shoulder movements and elevation and depression of the shoulder girdle elevation and depression are used). Repeat movements 20/50/75/100 times or as you can **(Figures 22.48 and 22.49)**.

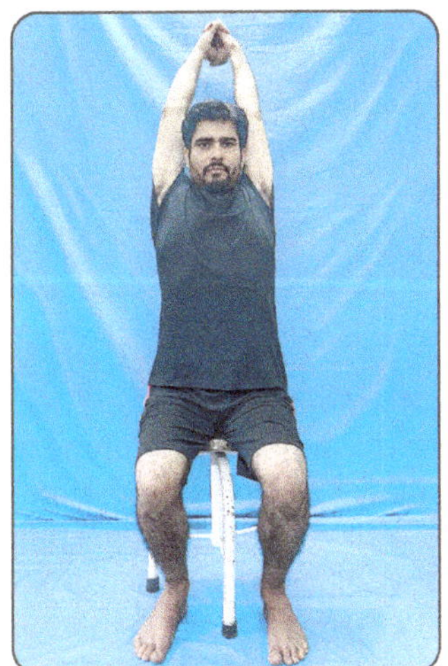

FIG. 22.48: NVY

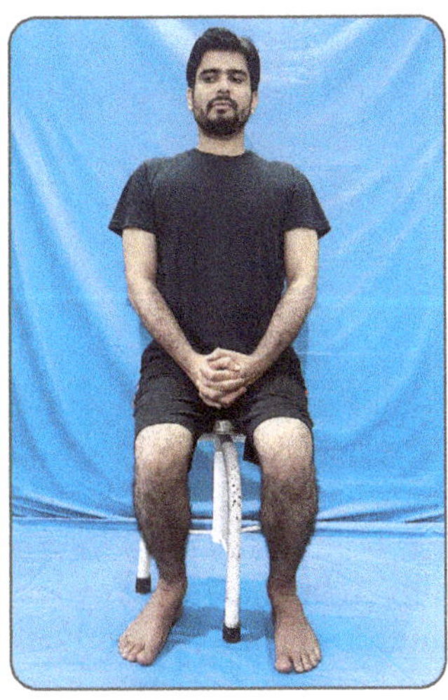

FIG. 22.49: NVY

8. In shoulder exercise rotatory movements are mandatory to be improved. These are very much helpful to prevent and treat adhesive capsulitis. Rotatory movements of shoulder should be done with elbows flexed to 90° (as in **Figures 22.50 and 22.51**) and elbows extended **(Figures 22.52 and 22.53)**

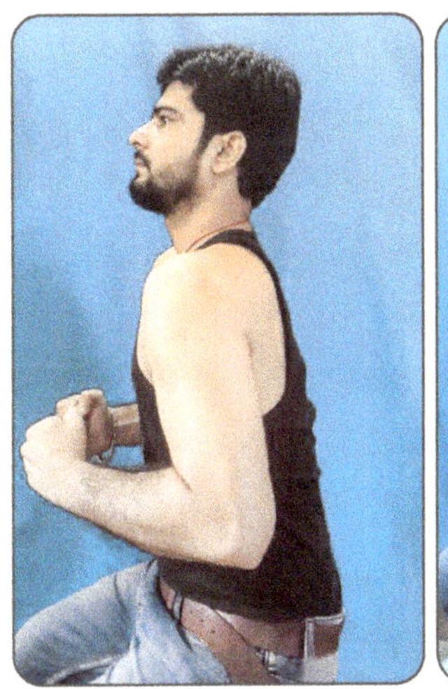

FIG. 22.50: NVY

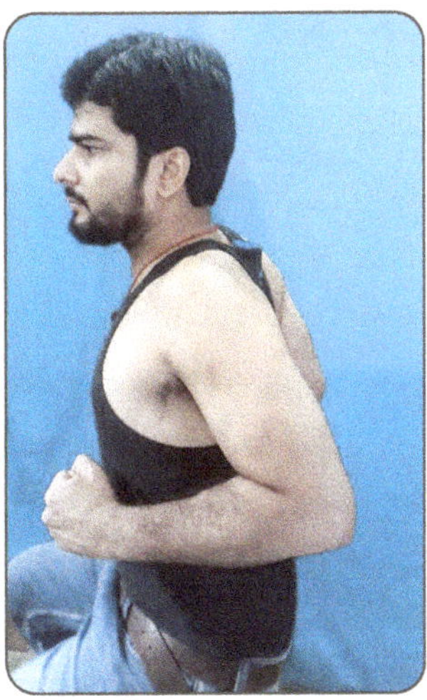

FIG. 22.51: NVY

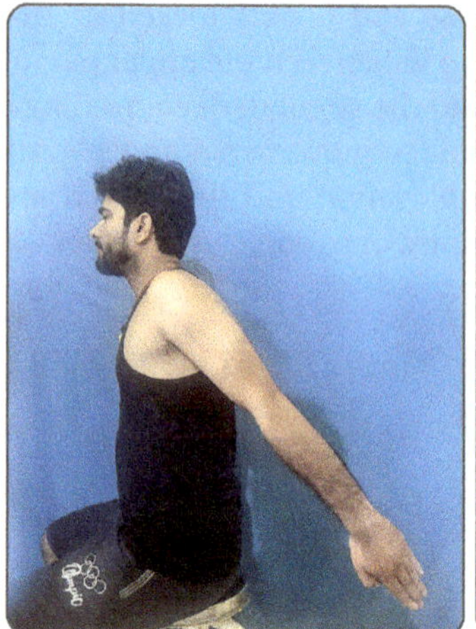

FIG. 22.52: NVY

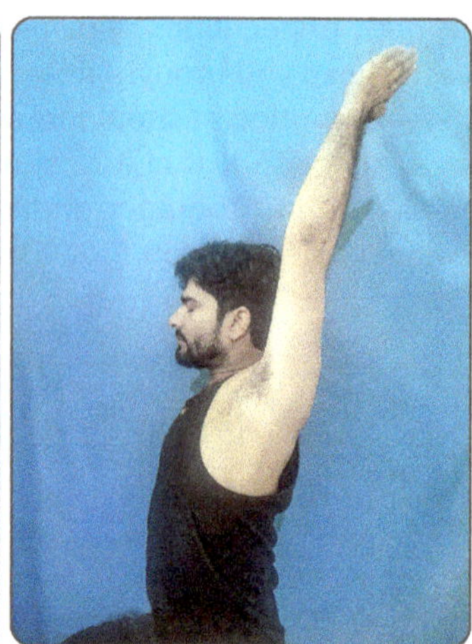

FIG. 22.53: NVY

Actions: Sit erect on the chair, arms should be closed to the chest now rotatory movements complete to be done anteroposterior and posteroanterior directions to full range (or as much as possible).

9. Sit erect, hold both hands through tight extended fingers, abduct both shoulders simultaneously as far as possible and sustained in this position for about 20 seconds bring back the arms closed to the chest repeat this maneuver 50–100 times it improves the abduction of shoulder and clears any residual adhesions of shoulder joint. Rotatory movements of the shoulder should be done with elbow straight making a full circle at the site of check. Semi rotation can be done with elbow flexed above 90°, holding the hand rail of walker tightly which will provide stability in erect position then stretched vertically as much as possible **(Figures 22.54 and 22.55)**. Sustain in this position for 20 seconds, then come down with

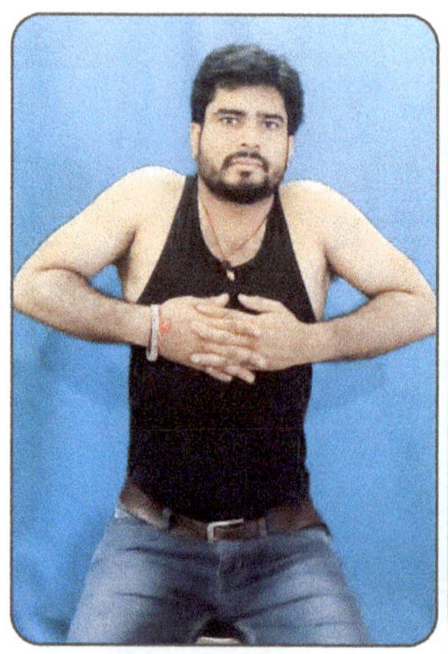

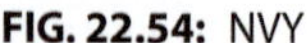

FIG. 22.54: NVY

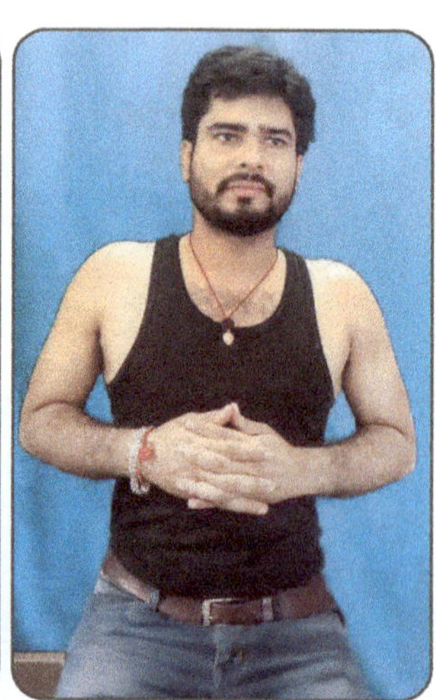

FIG. 22.55: NVY

toes touching the floor, repeat this process 50–100 times or as much as possible. It has been found that most of the Nakh Sikh yoga position can be performed in lying down position, as well.

10. a. Elevation of shoulder stretch the upper limbs forward fully and move palms alternately toward the earth and sky, repeat it 50–100 times **(Figures 22.56 and 22.57)**.

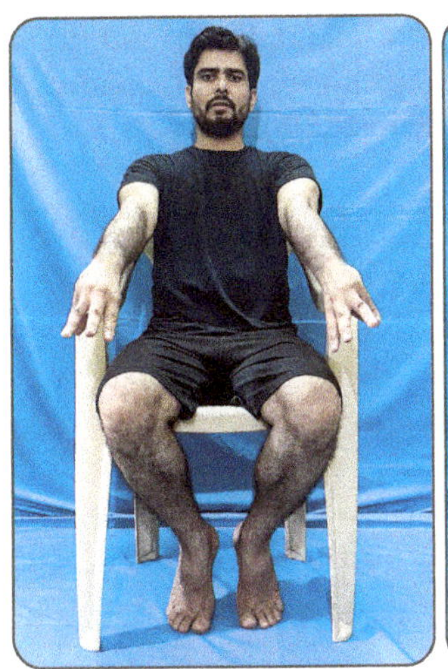

FIG. 22.56: NVY

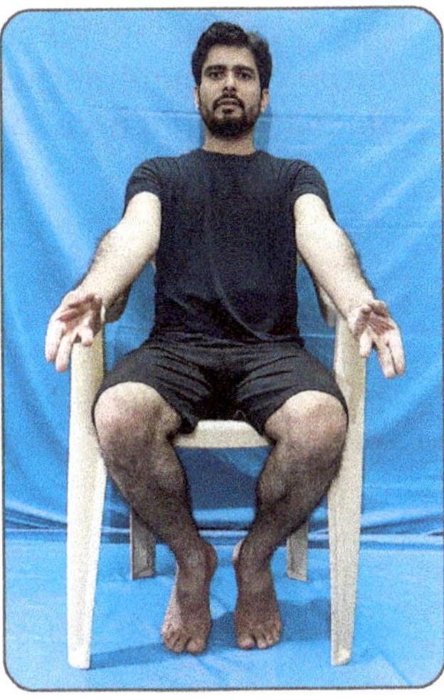

FIG. 22.57: NVY

b. In the same position of upper limbs make firm fists and open the fingers fully, repeat it 50–100 times.

c. In the same position of upper limbs open the fingers and thumbs fully—touch the tip of fingers by the tip of thumbs in succession 50–100 times **(Figures 22.58 and 22.59)**. Buddhi mudra, this yoga strengthens the intuitive knowledge.

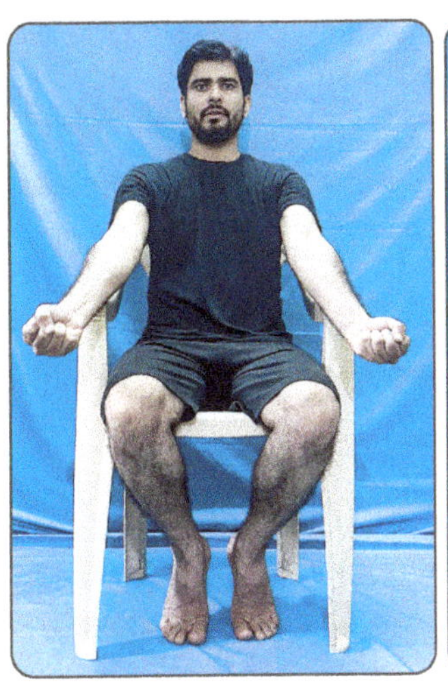

FIG. 22.58: NVY

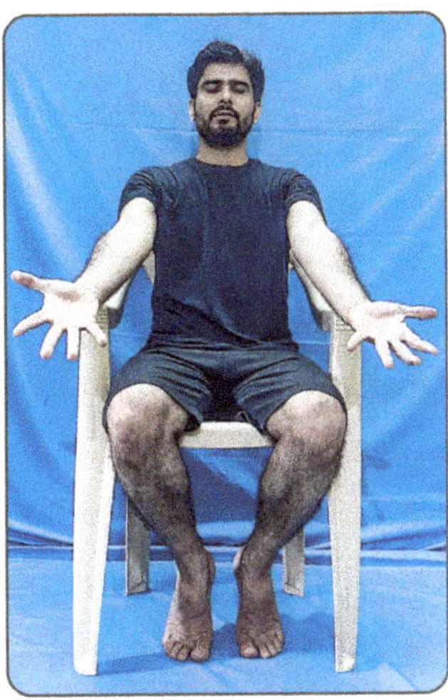

FIG. 22.59: NVY

i. In this maneuver, the supination and pronation of forearms, and varying extent of external and internal rotators of shoulders get improved.

ii. The firm fisting and opening up the fingers make them strong and useful to full extent.

iii. Thumb is said to be half hand, and its main action is probably the apposition, which accentuates the utility of other movements. Hence special attention on maintaining and improving all functions of thumb-including opposing and rotatory movements is mandatory **(Figures 22.60 to 22.65)**.

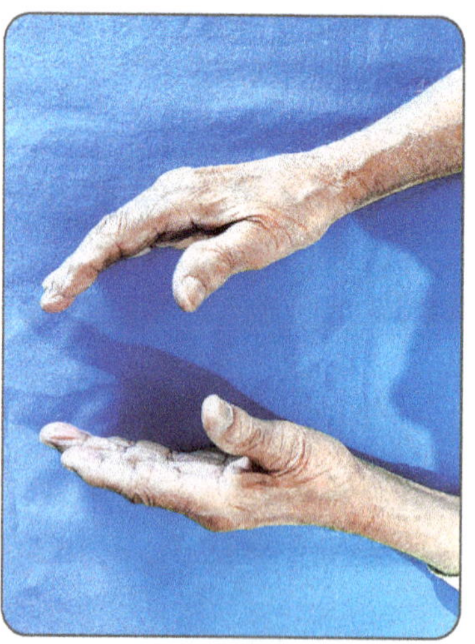

FIG. 22.60: NVY

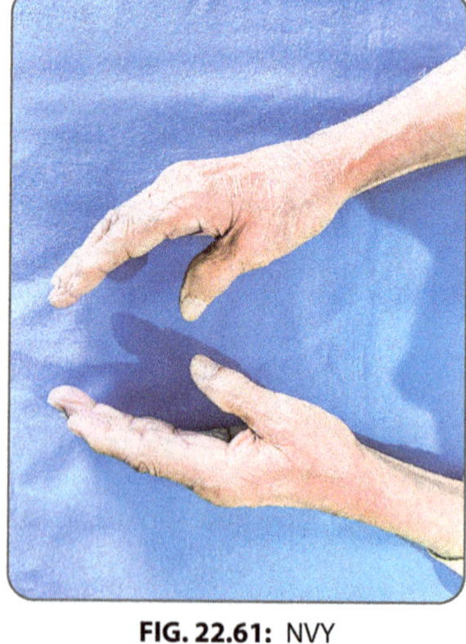

FIG. 22.61: NVY

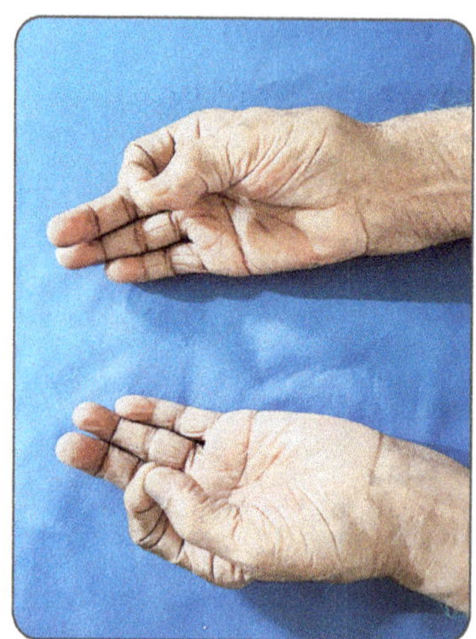

FIG. 22.62: NVY

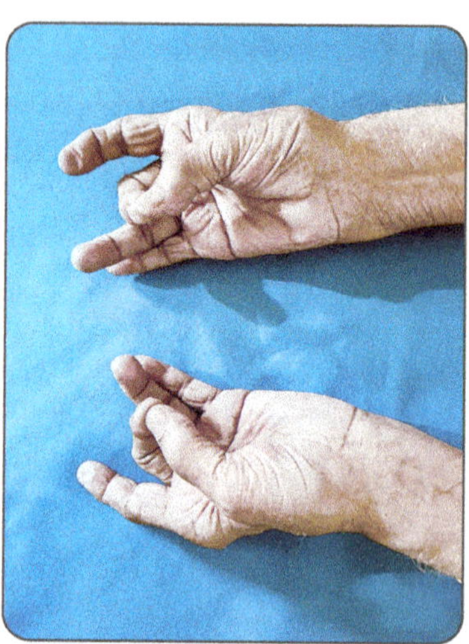

FIG. 22.63: NVY

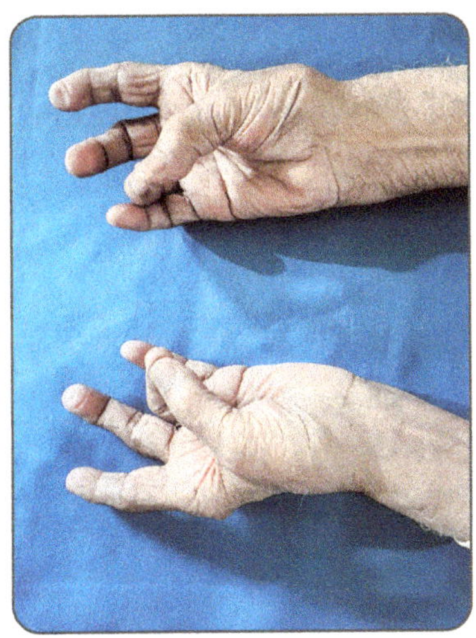

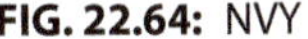

FIG. 22.64: NVY

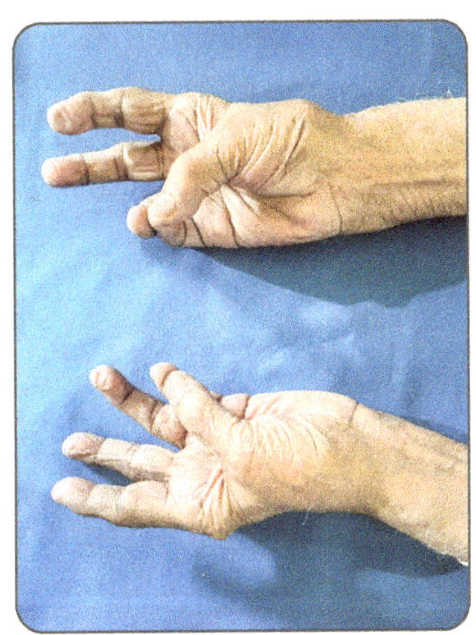

FIG. 22.65: NVY

11. Sit erect keeping the opened up palm of one hand on the same side ear and the opposite side opened up hand on that side iliac crest or knee. Now press the hands at their respective points and along with elevate the chest, sustain the position for 5–10 seconds repeat the process, and repeat the whole position to 50–100 times, or as much as you can on regular basis **(Figure 22.66)**

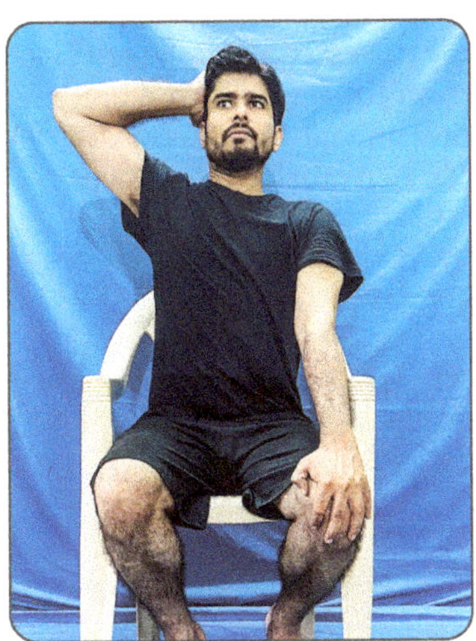

FIG. 22.66: NVY

Repeat the same process by changing the hands for the other sides. For keeping the head up and erect the power of neck muscles must be properly improved.

12. Firmly support the chin on the proximal parts of both palms. Keeping the neck tight, press the chin on the palms for about 5–10 to 20 seconds and then release it. Alternately do this process 50–100 times **(Figure 22.67)**.

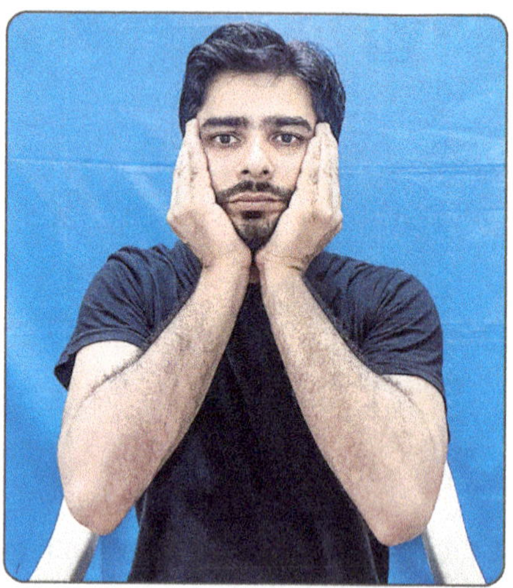

FIG. 22.67: NVY

The flexing of head for any work or looking down, the flexors of neck must be strong, which can be improved by the above exercises. To keep the head erect the extensors of the neck must be improved, for which the exercises noted as below are very helpful.

13. Sit with body and neck erect at the edge of couch—take both hands with locked fingers on the back of head and press the occipital region and maintain the pressure for 10–20 seconds—Release the pressure, and repeat the process 50–100 times **(Figure 22.68)**.

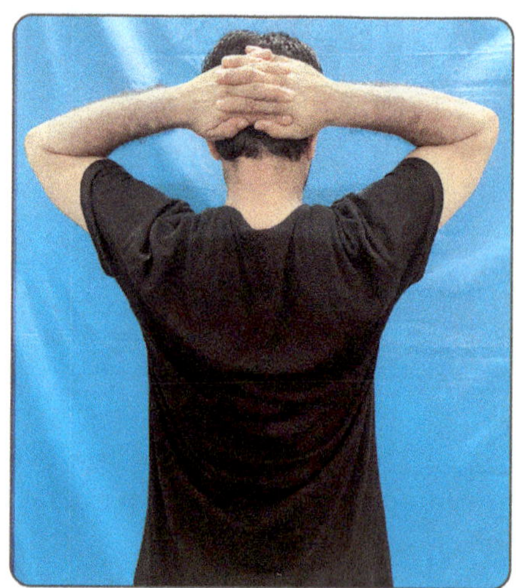

FIG. 22.68: NVY

14. **Butterfly exercises:** Lying flat on bed flex the hips by 70° to 80°, abduct the hips by about 60°, keep the knees flexed by 90°, and ankles plantar-flexed by 40° and soles adapted to each other. Bring the knees as much as possible to midline, and then take the knees back on bed—repeat the process like wings of butterfly **(Figure 22.69)**.

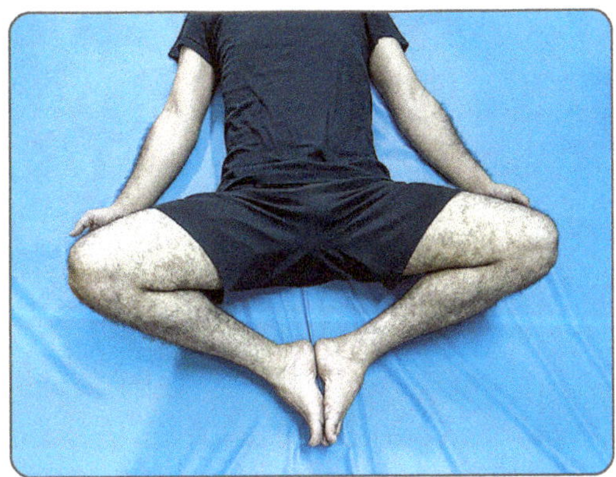

FIG. 22.69: NVY

In butterfly exercises, except extension of the hip other movements are practiced to the varying extent. With repeated actions the range of motions are made smooth and power of concerned muscles improved.

15. **For Eyes:** Sit erect at the edge of couch—Fix the opened eyes **(Figure 22.70)** in the front on any object/picture (better any religious picture) for about 10 seconds then close the eyes squeezing **(Figure 22.71)** the eyelids fully. Repeat opening and closing (for 10+10 seconds cycle). Do it 100 times. Now open up the eyes fully—elevate and depress the eyebrows alternately 50 times.

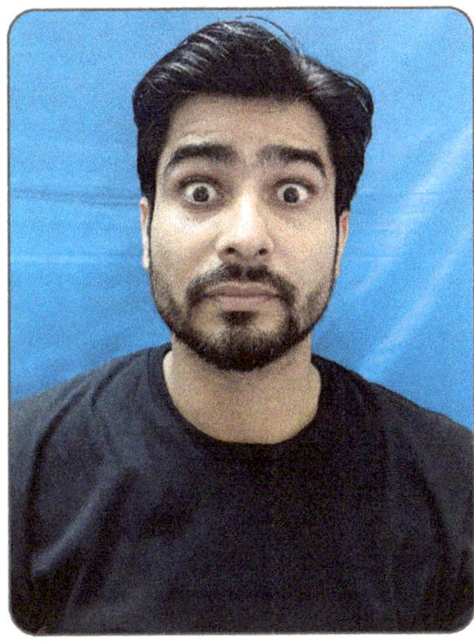

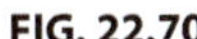

FIG. 22.70

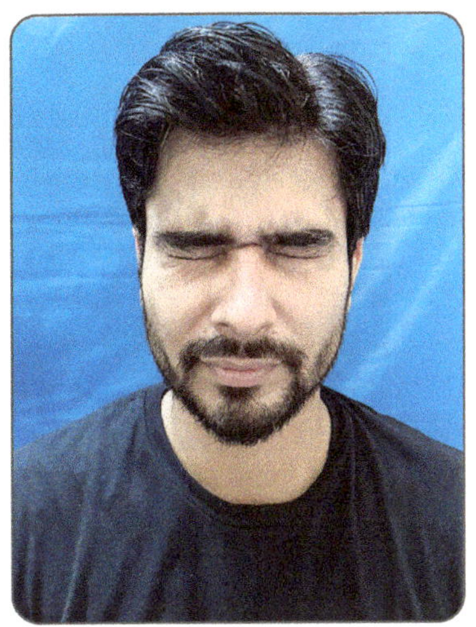

FIG. 22.71

Take the eyeballs to extreme right then to extreme left **(Figures 22.72 and 22.73)**.

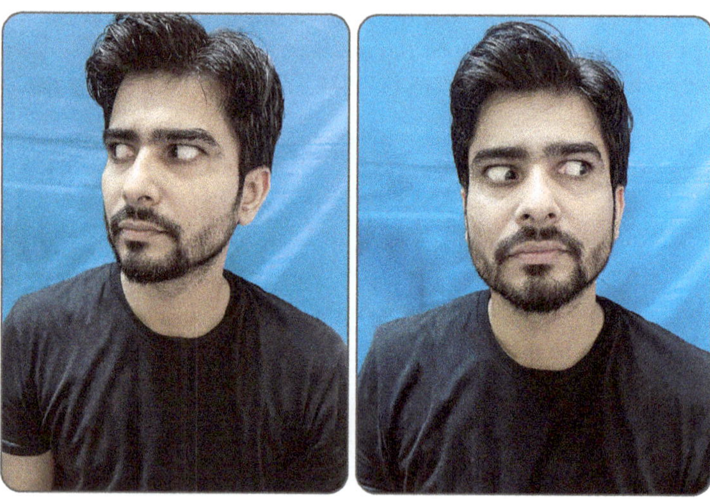

FIG. 22.72 **FIG. 22.73**

Open up the eyes fully—rotate eyeballs in clockwise and anticlockwise 50 times each.

The protection of eyeball is much important to avoid any overuse and any injury to them. The exercises of eyelids taking them upwards and downwards alternately are also essential **(Figures 22.74 and 22.75)**.

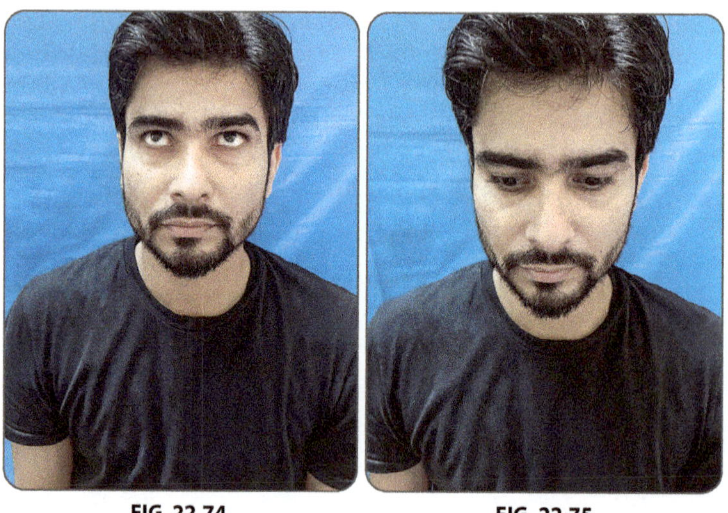

FIG. 22.74 **FIG. 22.75**

5 Yoga Poses to Prevent Obesity

Trikonasana
– Triangle pose

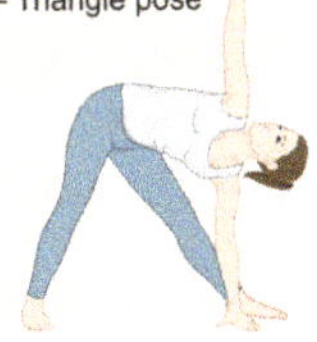

- **Reduce** the fat deposited in the **belly** and **waist**
- **Accelerates blood** flow throughout the body
- **Build muscles** in thighs and hamstrings
- Helps to **improve** digestion
- **Enhances** balance and focus

Parivrtta utkatasana
– Twisted chair pose

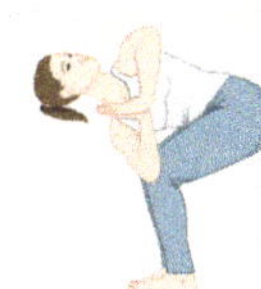

- **Stimulates** abdominal organs
- Advances **core muscles** and **core strength**
- **Improves** the **lymph system** and the **digestive system**
- **Increase** muscle **tone** and **strength**

Sethu bandha sarvangasana
– Bridge pose

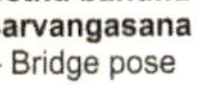

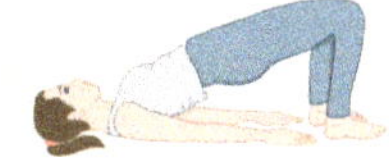

- **Regulates hormones** and **improves thyroid** levels
- **Strengthens** back muscles and **reduces** back pain
- Helps to **improve digestion** and **muscle tone**
- **Reduces hypertension** and **menopause** symptoms

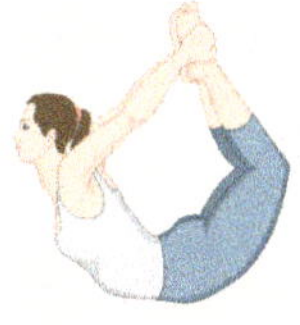

Dhanurasana
– Bow pose

- **Strengthens muscles** of thighs, chest, and back
- **Massage** abdominal organs
- Gives relief from **digestive problems**
- Alleviates **stress** and **anxiety** levels

Adho mukha svanasana
– Downward dog pose

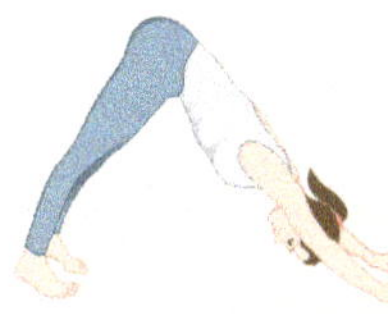

- **Increases** the **blood flow** to facial region that helps in **flushing out toxins** and **treating acne**
- **Improve immunity** and **keep healthy** from the inside out
- **Strengthens** and **tones** the upper body
- Instant **stress busting** effects

Postmenopausal Yoga Poses
Supine spinal twist
Snail
Pigeon
Balasana
Legs up the wall

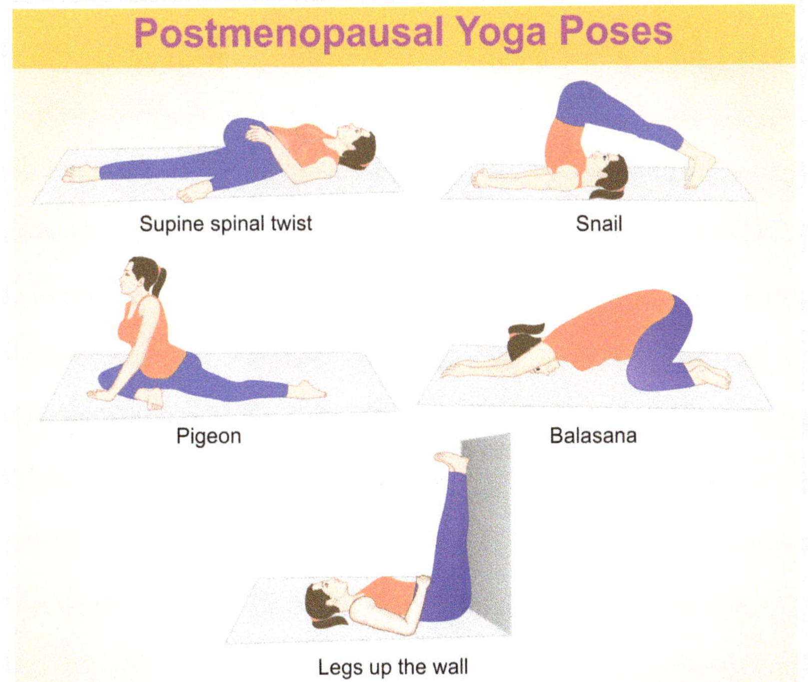

classic india
Kuchipudi

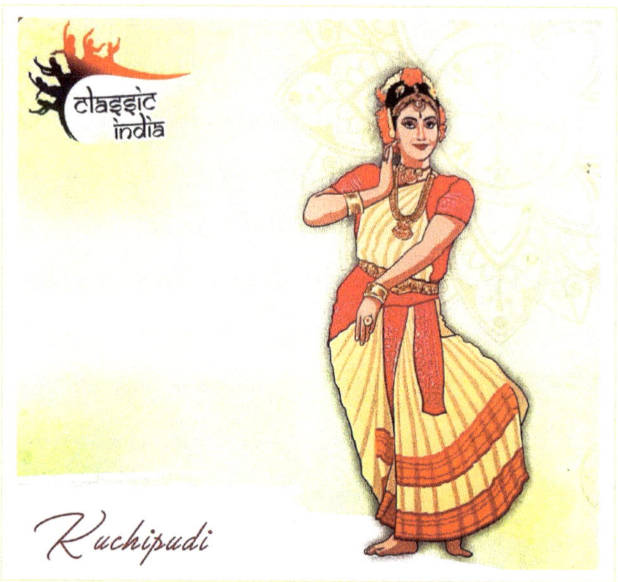

Classical Indian dances summarise most of the yoga poses and prove very much helpful in preventing obesity and improve the agility of body.

classic india
Lavani
One of the most popular folk dances of Maharashtra is 'Lavani.' Lavani is known for its energic movements and captivating music. This dance form, performed by a group of female dancers, combines rhythmical footwork, expressive gestures, and soulful singing. The lyrics of Lavani often revolve around love, society, and contemporary issues, making it a form of social commentary. The vibrant costumes adorned by the dancers, comprising colorful sarees with exquisite jewelry, add to the visual spectacle of the performance.

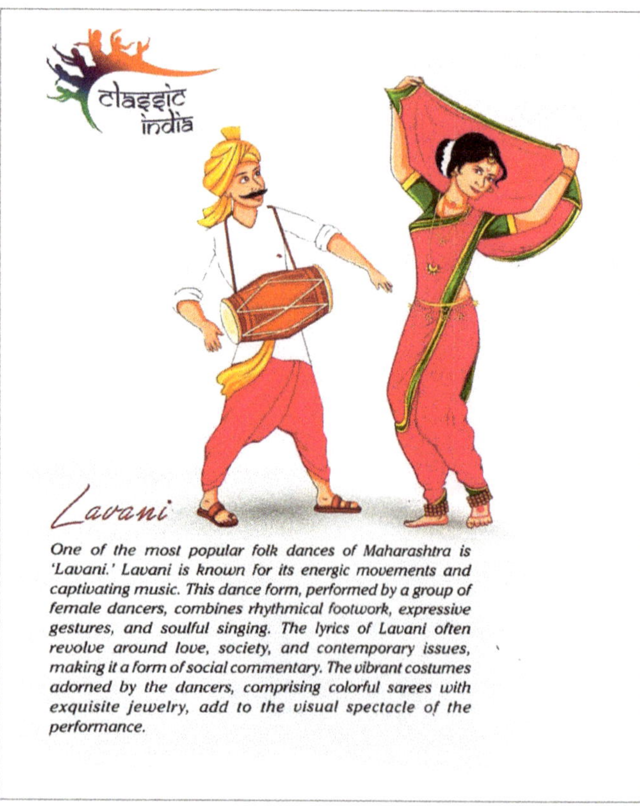

Appendices

Appendix 1

HISTORY OF MATERIALS USED FOR INTRA-ARTICULAR INJECTION

S. No.	Worker	Year	Materials used for intra-articular injection	Remarks
1.	*Koning*	1932	*Iodized oil*	
2.	*Thomson*	1933	*Pregl's solution of iodine* with sodium bicarbonate and Sodium chloride in watery solution	
3.	*Key*	1933	Claimed to have produced experimental osteoarthritis with intra-articular injection of weak acids, alkalies, distilled water and salt solution. These solutions were later utilized as theraputic measures by Koning Thomson and Andernach	All these were small series with slender theoretical basis and so were denied general acceptance
4.	*Andernach and Lohr*	1936	*Pure liver injections*	
5.	*Waugh*	1936 1938 1945	• *Lactic acid with procaine at pH 5* • He claimed good results in osteoarthritis, traumatic arthritis and rheumatoid arthritis. Discovering the identical pH of synovial fluid to that of blood, i.e., 7.4–7.6. Waugh propounded his acidification thereby. He suggested that acidity excites a polymorphonuclear leucocytosis followed later by local metablastic proliferation and this helps in clinical improvement. He further suggested that the change in pH helped to nourish the cartilage better. Acidification theory stimulated other workers who used lactic acid	
6.	*Crowe*	1944	*Acid potassium phosphate*	
7.	*Kron*	1948	*Sodium bicarbonate*	Encouraging results

Continued

Continued

S. No.	Worker	Year	Materials used for intra-articular injection	Remarks
8.	*Lawther*	1949	Lactic acid and procaine solution Procaine hydrochloride solution alone	Observed equal results
9.	*Melkid*	1953	Procaine alone	
10.	*Ross Mayer and Shepherd*	1958	*Benzyl salicylate*	
11.	*Desmarais*	1952	1. *Alkaline procaine solution* at pH 7.4 marked difference in these groups 2. Normal saline pH 7.2 *Waugh's acidification theory* 3. Mock injections 4. *Waugh's lactic acid*, procaine pH 5.4	Did not find any Did not support
12.	*Baker and Chayen*	1948	*Lactic acid in 2% procaine* (pH 5.4) 0.5% procaine adjusted to pH 7.6 with sodium phosphate normal saline	The results in the different series were almost identical, hence, they claimed that acid solution produced no benefit compared to those of physiological pH
13.	*Scott*	1943	10% Benzyl salicylate in oil	Observed good result in osteoarthritis and other rheumatoid disorder
14.	*Elkin*	1945	10% *Benzyl salicylate in oil*	Observed encouraging results
15.	*Broadman*	1954	10% Benzyle salicylate in oil	
16.	*Von Reis and Swenson*	1951	Osmic acid in animals and painful joint of human beings	Noticed widespread
17.	*Shutkin*	1951	Intra-articular nitrogen mustard to effect *chemical synovectomy* without causing cartilage damage	Mitchell, Laurin Shepard (1973) contraindicated the utility of *osmic acid* and *nitrogen mustards* for effecting *chemical synovectomy* as these chemicals were subsequently noticed to cause disintegration of cartilage surface
18.	*Scherbel, Shuciter and Weyman*	1957	Same as (17)	

Continued

Continued

S. No.	Worker	Year	Materials used for intra-articular injection	Remarks
18.	*Scherbel, Shuciter and Weyman*	1957	Same as (17)	
19.	*Makin and Robin*	1964	Intra-articular *radioactive gold* for treating chronic synovial effusions	
20.	*Chacha, Karim*	1978	Intra-articular papain, acetyl salicylic acid indomethacin, prostaglandin and alcohol	Experimental study to produce a good experimental model of osteoarthritis
21.	*Thorn (Quoted by Hollander 1951)*	1950	*Compound 'F' (hydrocortisone)*	Intra-articular injection into rheumatoid Observed encouraging results
22.	*Hollander, Brown, Jessar and Brown*	1951	Compound (F)	Intra-articular injection into inflamed knee Prompt alleviation of local effect
23.	*Freyberg et al. (Quoted by Hollander et al. 1951)*	1951	Cortisone	Intra-articular into knee joint
24.	*Mason et al. (Quoted by Hollander 1951)*	1951	Preferred hydrocortisone to cortisone for injection	
25.	*Miller, White and Morton*	1958 1958	To determine the true status of certain intra-articular injections used lactic acid, navocaine any significant *hydrocortisone acetate* with controls of physiological normal saline and mock injections	They did not find different series. They suggested the possibilities of physiological implications following injection
26.	*Feffer*	1965	• Intra-discal injection of hydro-cortisone in patients having backache • Rest either had no initial response or the patients had presented with recurrences • He inferred that older age group patients having primarily only backache without any radicular affection and having limited degenerative changes of involved sufficiency well	47.6% patients responded
27.	*Mukherjee K*	1982	Acetyl salycylic acid 2% pH 4.4	Under trial

Appendix 2

DISEASE MODIFYING OSTEOARTHRITIS DRUGS

Approval of Disease-modifying osteoarthritis drugs (DMOADs) in management of OA of hip and knee and also in rheumatoid arthritis has manifested relevant symptomatic benefits. They are:

1. *Repurposing existing triamcinolone*, which maintains the concentration this repurposed drug in joint for several months after the single dose and claims to provide greater pain relief in 5–10 weeks.
2. *Small molecule inhibition of Wnt signaling pathway (Wingless-related integration site).*
3. *Intra-articular small molecule BNTA effective* has also claims to be effective in OA knee. It promotes cartilage extracellular matrix generation thereby inhibiting further osteoarthritis development.
4. *Intra-articular stem cell (stem one)*: It is adult human bone marrow derived, cultured, pooled, allogenic mesenchymal stromal cells on vehicle hyaluronic acid. It claims effectiveness for stage II and early stage III OA.
5. *Intra-articular gene therapy* has been approved by US FDA in 2017. This futuristic first arthritis gene therapy is delivered in vivo by direct intra-articular injections.
6. *Sprifermin recombinant fibroblast growth factor-18 (FGF18)* in intra-articular foreword trail has showed to increase cartilage thickness, substantially reduces cartilage loss and its structural benefits may be seen at year 2 and sustained at year 5.
7. *Intra-articular injections in pipeline*:
   a. Botox
   b. Capsaicin
   c. Low molecular weight—human serum albumin
   d. Tenezubzm III—nerve growth factor

By the courtesy of
Prof (Dr) SS Jha

Bibliography

1. Adams ME, Atkinson MH, Lussier AJ, et al. The role of viscosupplementation with Hylan G-F 20 (Synvisc) in the treatment of osteoarthritis of the knee: A Canadian multicenter trial comparing hylan G-F 20 alone, Hylan G-F 20 with non-steroidal anti-inflammatory drugs (NSAIDs) and NSAIDs alone. Osteoarthritis Cartilage. 1995;3:213-25.
2. Ambra LF, Girolamo LD, Mosier B, Gomoll AH. Review: Interventions for Cartilage Disease: Current State-of-the-Art and Emerging Technologies. Arthritis Rheumatol. 2017;69(7):1363-73.
3. Andereoh F, Lohr W. ZBI Chir. 1936;63:2493.
4. Anderson DJ Gage FH, Weissman IL. Can stem cells cross linage boundaries? Nat Med. 2001;7:393-5.
5. Baker DM, Chayen MS. Treatment of arthritis, by intra-articular injection. Lancet. 1948; 1:93.
6. Balasz EA, Denlinger JL. Viscosupplementation: A new concept in the treatment of osteoarthritis. J Rheumatol. 1993;20(Suppl 39):3-9.
7. Balazs EA, Bloom GD, Swann DA. Fine structure and glycosaminoglycan content of the surface layer of articular cartilage. Fed Proc. 1966;25:1813-16.
8. Balazs EA, Freeman MI, Kloti R, Meyer-Schwickerath G, Regnault F, Sweeney DB. Hyaluronic acid replacement of vitreous and aqueous humor. Mod Probl Ophthalmol. 1972:10:3-21.
9. Balazs EA. The physical properties of synovial fluid and the special role of hyaluronic acid. In: Helfet A (Ed): Disorders of the knee. Philadelphia: Lippincott. 1974, pp. 61-74.
10. Balazs EA. Viscoelastic properties of hyaluronic acid and biological lubrication. (Symposium: Prognosis for Arthritis: Rheumatology Research Today and Prospects for Tomorrow, Ann Arbor, Michigan, 1967). Univ Mich Med Civ J. 1968;(Suppl): 255-59.
11. Barr JD, Barr MS, Lemley TJ, et al. Percutaneous vertebroplasty for pain relief and spinal stabilization. Spine. 2000;25:923-8.
12. Broadman J. J Med Sec N J. 1954;51:320.
13. Buchowski JM Adowa O. What's new in spine surgery. J Bone Joint Surg Am. 2019;101:1043-9.
14. Careette S, Moffet H, Tardif J, et al. Intra-articular corticoids, supervised physiotherapy or a combination of the two in the treatment of adhesive capsulitis of the shoulder: A placebo-controlled trial. Arthritis Rheum. 2003;48:829-838.
15. Carroll JE, Mays RW. Update on stem cell therapy for cerebral palsy. Expert Opin Biol Ther. 2011;11:463-71.
16. Chadha M, Agrawal A, Arora A. The Stem Cells in Orthopedic Surgery. In: Kulkarni GS, Babhulkar S (Eds). Textbook of Orthopedics and Trauma, 3rd Edition. Jaypee Brothers Medical Publishers; 2016. pp. 47-51.
17. Chen G, Wang Y, Xu Z, Fang F, Xu R, Wang Y, et al. Neural Stem Cell like cells derived from autologous bone mesenchymal stem cells for the treatment of patients with cerebral palsy. J Transl Med. 2013;11:21.
18. Crowe HW. In Octavio Calvillo, Ioannis Skaribas, Joseph Turnipseed (Eds): Treatment of arthritis with acid potassium phosphate. Lancet. 1944;1:563.
19. Deepak KK, Rao MR. Yoga and Meditation as an Adjunct Interventional Strategy for COVID-19 Management. Ann Natl Acad Med Sci (India). 2021;57:65-67.
20. Desmarais MHL. Value of intra-articular injection in osteoarthritis. Annals of the Rheumatoid Disease. 1952;11:277.

21. Elkin AC. Med Press. 1945;213:350.
22. Eustace JA, Brophy DP, Gibney RP, et al. Comparison of the accuracy of steroid placement with clinical outcome in patients with shoulder symptoms. Ann Rheu Dis. 1997;56: 59-63.
23. Feffer HL. Therapeutic intra-discal hydrocortisone: A long term evaluation study and analysis. J Bone and Join Surg. 1965;47:1287.
24. Friedenstein AJ, Petrakova KV, Kurolesova AI, Frullova GP. Heterotopic of bone marrow. Analysis of precursor cells for osteogenic and hematopoietic tissues. Transplantation. 1968;6:230-47.
25. Friedenstein AJ, Piatelzky SII, Petrakova KV. Osteogenesis in transplants of bone marrow cells. J Embryol Exp Morphol. 1966;16:381-90.
26. Friedman DM, Moore ME. The efficacy of intra-articular steroids in osteoarthritis: A double-blind study. J Rheumatol. 1980;7:850-6.
27. Gaffney K, Ledingham, Perry JD. Intra-articular triamcinolone hexacetonide in knee osteoarthritis: Factors influencing the clinical response. Ann Rheum Dis. 1995;54: 379-81.
28. Goodman LS, Gilman A. The pharmacological basis of therapeutic (5th edn). New York: Macmillan Publishing Company Inc. 1975;1987-88.
29. Gulefi M, Pantalone A, Vanni D, et al. Long-term beneficial effects of platelet-rich plasma for non-insertional Achilles tendinopathy. Foot Ankle Surg. 2015;21:178-81.
30. Helfet AJ. Management of osteoarthritis of the knee joint. In: Helfet (Ed). Disorders of the knee. Philadelphia: JB Lippincott Co. 1974;175-94.
31. Hollander JL, Brown Jr, Jessar RA, Brown CY. Hydrocortisone and cortisone injected into arthritic joints. J Arm Med Assn. 1951;147:1629.
32. Hollander JL, Jessar RA, Brown EM Jr. Intrasynovial corticosteroid therapy: A decade of use. Bulletin of Rheumatic Diseases. 1961;11:239.
33. Hollander JL. Ann Inter Med. 1953;39:735.
34. Hue AG, Rkain H, Abdul mutalib, et al. The place of platelet-rich plasma in Traumatic in and Degenerative diseases of the foot and ankle. Literature review. Foot Medicine and Surgery. 2016;32–4:102-8.
35. Hyashi T, Furukawa H, Funayama, et al. A new uniform protocol of combined corticosteroid injections and ointment application reduce recurrence rates after surgical keloid/hypertrophic scar excision. Dermatol Surg. 2012;38(6):893-7.
36. James A, Doherty M, et al. Intra-articular corticosteroids are effective in osteoarthritis but there are no clinical predictors of response. Ann Rheum Dis. 1996;55:829-32.
37. Jayavelu P, Sambandar T. Medical treatment modalities of oral submucous fibrosis. NJIRM. 2012;3(2):147-51.
38. Jha SS. Observations on the effects of repeated intra-articular injections of hydro-cortisone acetate: An experimental study. Thesis for the Master of Surgery (Orthopaedics) Ranchi University, 1978.
39. Johansson A, Hao J, Sjolund B. Local corticosteroid application blocks transmission in normal nociceptive C-fibres. Acta Anaesthesiol Seand. 1990;34:335-8.
40. Karak M, Ugras S, Tosun N, et al. The effects of intra-articular administration of hyaluronan and cortisone in the rabbit's knee: A comparative experimental study with histopathologic evaluations. Orthopaedic Update (India). 2001;II(2):68-71.
41. Kashyap A -HOD Cosmetology at Fortis La Femme-Published in the Pioneer daily Newspaper on 27/05/2008.
42. Key JA. Production of chronic arthritis by the injection of weak acids, alkalies, distilled water and salt solution into joints. J Bone Joint Surg. 1939;15:67.
43. Kim DJ, Yun YH, Wang JM. Nerve-root injections for the relief of pain in patients with osteoporotic vertebral fractures. J Bone Joint Surg. 2003;85-B:250-3.
44. Koing W. Zbl Chir. 1930;59:1907.

45. Kolasinski SL, Neogi T, Hochberg MC, Oatis C, Guyatt G, Block J, et al. 2019 American College of Rheumatology/Arthritis Foundation Guideline for the Management of Osteoarthritis of the Hand, Hip, and Knee. Arthritis Rheumatol. 2020;72(2):220-33.
46. Kron R. Die intra-articular-alkali—Therapic schweizer ische medizinesche wochenschrift. 1948;78:80.
47. Kumar S. A randomized control study comparing the Efficacy of Triamcinolone injection versus Platelet- Rich Plasma in Rotator Cuff Tendinopathy. IOACON 2019, Abstract Book, p. 97.
48. Kumar V, Siwach K. Comparison of periarticular local infiltration versus Buprenorphine Transdermal Patch for pain management and Rehabilitation in Total hip and Knee arthroplasty Patients. IOACON 2019, Abstract Book Kolkata, p.128.
49. Laird H. Ozone Injections Promising in Knee Osteoarthritis. November 13, 2015 in Highlights from ACR 2015 San Francisco11-17 Nov 2015.
50. Lavelle ED, Lavelle L, Intraarticular injections. Med Clin N An. 2007;91:241-50.
51. Lavelle W, Lavelle ED, Lavelle L. Intra-articular Injections. Anesthesiology Clin. 25 (2007); 853-62.
52. Lawther K. Ann Rheum Dis. 1948;8:178.
53. Lee KT, Kim JS, Young KW, Lee YK, Park YU, Kim YH, et al. The use of fibrin matrix-mixed gel-type autologous chondrocyte implantation in the treatment for osteochondral lesions of the talus. Knee Surg Sports Traumatol Arthrosc. 2013;21(6):1251-60.
54. Lim JK, Hui J, Li L, Thambyah A, Goh J, Lee EH. Enhancement of tendon graft osteointegration ligament reconstruction. Arthroscope. 2004;20(9);899-910.
55. Mahindra P, Yamin M, Sethi, et al. Chronic plantar fascitis: effect of platelet-rich plasma, corticosteroid and placebo. Orthopaedics. 2016;39:285-9.
56. Mahowald ML, Singh JA, Dykstra D. Long term effects of intra-articular botulinum toxin A for refractory joint pain. Neurotox Res. 2006;9:179-88.
57. Makin M, Robin GC. Chronic synovial effusions treated with intra-articular radioactive gold. J American Medical Association. 1964;188:725.
58. Management of Osteoarthritis of the Knee (Non-Arthroplasty). Evidence-Based Clinical Practice Guideline. The American Academy of Orthopaedic Surgeons Board of Directors, 2021.
59. Meheux CJ, McCulloch PC, Linter DM, et al. Efficiency of intraarticular platelet-rich plasma injections in knee osteoarthritis; a systematic review. Arthroscopy. 2016;32: 495-505.
60. Melkid A. None Erfaringer Med procainbe handling Tidaskrift for den Norske Laegefor 1953;73:484.
61. Meretoja VV, Dahlin RL, Kasper FK, Mikos AG. Enhanced chondrogenesis in co-cultures with articular chondrocytes and mesenchymal stem cells. Biomaterials. 2012;33:6362-9.
62. Miller JH, White J, Morton TH. The value of intra-articular injections in osteoarthritis of the knee. J Bone and Joint Surg. 1958;403:636.
63. Namazi H. botulinum toxin as a novel addition to anti-arthritis armamentarium. An experimental study in rabbits. Intl Immunopharmacology. 2006:1743-7.
64. Namiki O, Toyoshima H, Morisaki N, Watnabe Y, Yamaguchi T. Studies on some properties of synovial fluid. Orthop Res Science. 1978;5:163-8.
65. Natarajan M. Trigeminal neuralgia-percutaneous trigeminal ganglion balloon compression. In hand bulletin of KG hospital, Coimbatore.
66. Octavio Calvillo, Ioannis Skaribas, Joseph Turnipseed. Anatomy and pathophysiology of the sacroiliac joint: Current Review of PAIN-(official publicator Lalorld Inscitute of Pain). Philadelphia: Current Science Inc. Panther Publishers Private Limited, Bangalore 2001; 12 to 17.
67. Patil SD, Patil VD, Luthra R, Ranaware A. Acute compartment syndrome of the foot due to infection after local hydrocortisone injection. J Foot Ankle Surg. 2015;54:692-96.

68. Pemberton R. Arthritis and rheumatoid conditions. Their nature and treatment. Philadelphia: Lea and Febiger; 1935.
69. Peyron JG. Intraarticular hyaluronan injections in the treatment of osteoarthritis. J Rheumatol. 1993;20:10-15.
70. Poro MA, Balasz EA, Belmote. Reduction of sensory responses to passive movements of inflamed knee joints by Hylan, a hyaluronan derivative. Exp Brain Res. 1997;Hb: 3-9.
71. Raynaud JP. Clinical trials: Impact of intra-articular steroid injections on the progression of knee osteoarthritis. Osteoarthritis Cartilage. 1999;7:348-9.
72. Raynauld JP, Buckland-Wright C, Ward R, et al. Safety and efficacy of intra-articular steroid injections on the progression of knee osteoarthritis: A randomized double-bind, placebo-controlled trial. Arthritis Rheum. 2003;48:370-7.
73. Reier PJ. Cellular transplantation strategies or spinal cord injury and transplantation neurobiology. NeuroRx. 2004;1(4):424-51.
74. Roman JA, Chismol J, Morales M, et al. Intraarticular treatment with hyaluronic acid. Comparative study of hyalgan and adant. Clin Reumatol. 2000;19:204-6.
75. Ropes MW, Bauer W. Synovial fuid changes in joint disease. Cambridge (MA): Harvard university press; 1953.
76. Ross KA, Mayer JH, Shepher MM. Osteoarthritis of the knee. Treatment by local injection of salicylate compounds. British Medical Journal. 1958;1:1040.
77. Rushing CJ, Rathnayake VR, Oxios AJ, Spinner SM, Hardigan P. Patient-Perceived Recovery and Outcomes after Bipolar Radiofrequency Controlled Ablation with Platelet-Rich Plasma Injection for Refractory Plantar Fasciosis. J Foot Ankle Surg. 2020;59(4):673-8.
78. Salvi AE. Targeting the plantar fascia for corticosteroid injection. The J Foot Ankle Surg. 2015;54:683-685.
79. Scherbel AL, Schueter SL, Weyman SJ. A rotational approach to the treatment of rheumatoid arthritis. Cleveland Clinic Quarterly. 1957;24:78.
80. Scott GL. British Med J. 1943;2:510.
81. Shetty SH, Dhond A, Arora M, Deore S. Platelet-Rich Plasma Has Better Long-Term Results Than Corticosteroids or Placebo for Chronic Plantar Fasciitis: Randomized Control Trial. J Foot Ankle Surg. 2019;58(1):42-6.
82. Shutkin NM. Note on the use of nitrogen mustard in rheumatoid arthritis. J Bone and Joint Surg. 1951;33:265.
83. Singh M, Gupta S, Rawat S, et al. Mechanisms of Action of Human Mesenchymal Stem Cells in Tissue Repair Regeneration and their Implications. Ann Natl Acad Med Sci (INDIA). 53(2);2017:104-20.
84. Singla A, Yang S, Werner BC, Cancienne JM, Nourbakhsh A, Shimer AL, et al. The impact of preoperative epidural injections on postoperative injection in lumber fusion surgery. J Neurosurg Spine. 2017;26(5);645-9.
85. Snibbe JC, Gambardella RA. Use of injections for osteoarthritis in joints and sports activity. Clin Sports Med. 2005;24(1):83-91.
86. Stiell (1922) Quoted by G. Andrew Murphy in 'Disorders of tendons and fascia and adolescent and adult pes planus'—In "Campbell's Operative Orthopaedics", Twelfth edition-Ediloss S terry canale James H Beaty, Elsevier Mosby; 2013: p3252.
87. Thomson JEM. Biophysical Journal. 1933;15:483.
88. Uthman I, Raynauld JP, Haraoui B. Intra-articular therapy in osteoarthritis. Postgrad Med J. 2003;79(934):449-53.
89. Venkatesan Nagarajan, et al. Low backache treatment with Botulinum Neurotoxin Type A Medical principal and practice, 2007;16:181-6.
90. Waugh WC. Treatment of certain joint lesions by injection of lactic acid. Lancet. 1938;1:487.
91. Waugh WG. Mono-articular osteoarthritis of the hip. British Medical Journal. 1945;1:873.
92. Xu J, Muhammad H, Wang X, Ma X. Botulinum Toxin type A injection combined with cast immobilization for treating recurrent peroneal spastic flat foot with bone coalitions: A case report and review of the literature. J Foot Ankle Surg. 2015;54:697-700.

Index

Page numbers followed by *f* refer to figure.

D

E

F

G

H

I

J

K

L

M

Q

R

S

T